Nursing Theories and Models

Nursing theory is a key element of all modern nursing courses, yet nurses are rarely encouraged to evaluate the models they are taught.

In *Nursing Theories and Models*, Hugh McKenna challenges the notion that certain nursing models are infallible, and examines strategies for bridging the gap between theory and practice. Readers are guided through the confusing terminology associated with nursing theory and are encouraged to test established models and assess the positive difference their use can have on patient care.

In addition to exploring the origins and abundance of current 'popular' models, the author examines whether new models should emanate from research, practice, or from other theories. He suggests that nurses themselves generate and select theories from their own practice, whether consciously or unconsciously, and that this skill can be developed through reflection and analysis.

Nursing Theories and Models is an essential text for students on both undergraduate and postgraduate nursing courses, and provides valuable insight for the practising professional into the strengths and weaknesses of the models they teach.

Hugh McKenna is a Senior Lecturer in Nursing at the University of Ulster and has written many books and articles on nursing theory.

Routledge Essentials for Nurses cover four key areas of nursing:

- core theoretical studies
- psychological and physical care
- nurse education
- new directions in nursing and health care

Written by experienced practitioners and teachers, books in this series encourage a critical approach to nursing concepts and show how research findings are relevant to nursing practice.

The series editors are **Robert Newell**, Lecturer in Nursing Studies, University of Hull and **David Thompson**, Professor of Nursing Studies, University of Hull.

Also in this series:

Nursing Perspectives on Quality of Life   Peter Draper
Teaching and Assessing Learners   Mary Chambers

Nursing Theories and Models

Hugh McKenna

London and New York

First published 1997
by Routledge
11 New Fetter Lane, London EC4P 4EE

Simultaneously published in the USA and Canada
by Routledge
29 West 35th Street, New York, NY 10001

Reprinted 1998, 2000

Routledge is an imprint of the Taylor & Francis Group

© 1997 Hugh McKenna

Typeset in Times by M Rules

Printed and bound in Great Britain by TJ International Ltd.,
Padstow, Cornwall

British Library Cataloguing in Publication Data
A catalogue record for this book is available from the British Library

Library of Congress Cataloguing in Publication Data
A catalogue record for this book has been requested

ISBN 0–415–14222–9 (hbk)   100224 7224
ISBN 0–415–14223–7 (pbk)

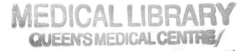

Contents

Illustrations

Boxes

Figures

Tables

Introduction

The knowledge base of a profession is normally expressed in the form of concepts, propositions and theories. Nursing has currently reached this level of theoretical evolution. This book will critically examine the development, selection, application and testing of nursing theories.

Just because practising nurses use nursing theories does not mean that they are theorising about nursing. Therefore, to enable nurses to understand the real importance of theory, the art and science of theorising will be discussed. The reader will be taken on a journey beginning with the identification of phenomena which are of interest to nursing through to conceptualising these phenomena in the form of propositions which can be analysed to form the building blocks of nursing theories.

In the mid-1980s nursing theories were introduced into most curricula and practice settings in Europe. In this regard nurses were following a trend set in the United States. The theories were very popular in the British nursing press and practising nurses were being encouraged to use them by educators and managers alike. In most cases, and with very little understanding as to what they were, nursing theories were applied, often without question, to a wide range of patient care settings. However, it was not immediately apparent what effect their study and use was having on the delivery and outcomes of patient care. One could ask, if nursing theories were as advantageous as reputed, why did most nurses have such a negative perception of them?

In essence, many nurses were brainwashed into believing that these theories held the answer, that they contained the essence of nursing. This was reinforced by the United Kingdom Central Council for Nursing, Midwifery and Health Visiting, which has voiced its support for nursing theories (Girot, 1990). In addition, Kershaw (1990) states that the DHSS 'Strategy for Nursing' takes as implicit that theory-based practice occurs. Cash (1990) went further by stating that theories are an explicit part of the curriculum for registered nurses.

Respected nursing leaders lent support to the introduction of nursing theories. According to Pearson (1986), a move toward theory-based practice was the most important target for change within nursing. Castledine (1986) believes that the implementation of a nursing theory leads to better nursing care and more reliable and critical observation by the nurse. Others wrote that the application of nursing theories to patient care would help improve the quality of the service delivered (Hardy, 1982; Farmer, 1986). Therefore, in many instances nursing theories were presented in the literature as a panacea for problems in nursing practice, education, management and research. However, few available research reports have confirmed the link between the use of a nursing theory and the quality of care delivered to or received by patients (McKenna, 1994a).

Until recently, criticism of these theories was actively discouraged; to criticise was to demonstrate that you were a laggard, a saboteur of change, an academic Luddite or, worse still, ignorant of these new conceptual initiatives. However, some nurses were worried at what appeared to be unsubstantiated acceptance and support. McFarlane (1986a), almost a lone voice, advocated that all nursing theories require careful analysis and evaluation in practice. Fawcett (1989) refers to this as 'credibility determination'. She states that credibility determination is necessary to avoid the uncritical acceptance of a nursing theory and to establish the effect of using a nursing theory on the outcomes of nursing care.

Yet, as we near the end of the twentieth century, a review of the literature reveals that such empirical information is conspicuous by its scarcity. As a result, there is little research evidence pertaining to the application, let alone the evaluation of nursing theories. None the less, contemporary nurses are beginning to have a healthy cynicism for nursing theories and are taking a more critical stance towards them. Analysing and evaluating these theories requires specific knowledge and skills, and nurses are increasingly being required to show such knowledge and skills.

The content of this book has its origins in the writer's teaching and research (McKenna, 1994a). Over a number of years, students, both at undergraduate and postgraduate levels, have stimulated the writer with their fresh views and critiques of nursing theories (McKenna, 1993). Practitioners too have contributed their opinions as to whether nursing theories were 'ideal' or 'real' (McKenna, 1992). There is the recognition that nurses throughout the world have spent an enormous amount of time and effort formulating, learning and implementing nursing theories. In the late 1990s it is perhaps time to suggest that 'the emperor has no clothes'. Therefore, the end result of these discussions, debates, arguments and reflections is a book which fills a niche in the market, one that uses the extant literature to provide a critical evaluation of nursing theories.

The proposed text differs from existing books on nursing theories in two respects. First, the focus is on exploring with the reader how theorising, analysis and testing should take place. Second, the conceptual basis is broader, taking a critical stance on the subject of nursing theories. It will be contended that real 'practitioner theorising' has been ignored in favour of 'off-the-shelf' theories. The humanistic, holistic and personal aspects of nurse conceptualising will be explored and realistic evaluative methodologies will be considered.

In the early chapters theories will be analysed in terms of their epistemological roots. The question of why they appeared in abundance in the mid-twentieth century will be addressed. Terminology will be explored and the various arguments surrounding the designations 'theory', 'model', 'paradigm' and 'framework' will be dissected. The borrowed versus home grown theory argument will be evaluated, as will the debate as to whether nursing can be a one-theory or multiple-theory profession.

The relationship between research and nursing theory will also be examined critically. There will be an exploration of the literature as to whether nursing theories emanate from research, from practice or from other theories. In addition, the testing of theories will be explored in detail, taking cognisance of the use of qualitative as well as quantitative approaches. Examples of theory testing of known nursing theories will be given.

A section will also be included relating to how educators, researchers and practitioners select nursing theories. The skills involved in this process will be analysed. Readers will be introduced to a comprehensive list of criteria that will enable them to judge the quality of nursing theories and how they affect the processes and outcomes of patient care.

To summarise, this book will give readers an insight into how practitioners theorise and how theories develop. The evolution of the many nursing theories we have today will be examined, taking into account why we have so many and whether one theory or many theories will continue to be our professional legacy. The role of research in theory generation will be analysed and how such theories may in turn guide future research.

Because there are so many nursing theories available to practitioners and academics, an in-depth exploration of selection strategies will be undertaken. Once aware of the pitfall of choosing appropriate theories, the reader will be encouraged to explore how these theories (or propositions within them) are tested by quantitative and qualitative research, or a triangulation of both. Because the plethora of nursing theories (forty-five) currently available to practitioners cannot all be inherently sound, rigorous frameworks for analysing and evaluating them will be presented.

Chapter 1
The trouble with terminology

Throughout our lives we are always learning new words and terms. For instance, 'compact disc', 'CD-ROM', 'greenhouse effect' and the 'Le Shuttle' are not terms which were familiar to our recent ancestors. Similarly, learning the rules of a new sport, starting a new job or taking up a hobby will bring with it a new set of terms. If we have sufficient interest we will spend some time learning the meaning of these new words.

The development of knowledge in nursing also brings with it new terms. These include 'theory', 'paradigm' and 'construct', to name just three. The same nurses who eagerly learn those new words associated with hobbies and sports often take an anti-intellectual stance when it comes to new words in nursing. This opening chapter proposes to introduce you to a range of terms which many readers may not have come across. My advice is that you look to the meaning behind the words and you will be richer for it.

While trawling the literature I have come across hundreds of definitions for the theoretical terms I will be addressing. I have noted that many definitions contradict each other and there is much disagreement among the experts. Therefore, it is highly probable that for each of the following definitions there is a contrary definition. I have attempted to get around this problem by selecting those definitions which have the most support in the literature.

I have categorised the terms into three groups. These are:

- Global terms
- Working terms
- Middle terms

Global terms

- Metaparadigm
- Domain
- Philosophy

Global terms are those expressions which represent a very broad view of issues that are relevant to nursing. A global view is like the view of a country from a satellite. The image is so all-encompassing that it is difficult to begin to describe the detail. None the less, this perspective is useful in that it provides you with a truly philosophic vantage-point.

Perhaps the best-known global term is 'metaparadigm'. This term is associated with the writings of Thomas Kuhn (1970), a philosopher, and Jacqueline Fawcett (1995), a nurse. According to Fawcett, a metaparadigm is:

> the most global perspective of a discipline acting as an encapsulating unit or framework within which the more restricted structures develop. It identifies certain phenomena which are of interest to a discipline and explains how that discipline deals with those phenomena in an unique manner.
>
> (Fawcett, 1992: 64)

Most authors subscribe to a four-component metaparadigm. These four components are: 'nursing', 'health', 'person', and 'environment' (Yura and Torres, 1975; Fawcett, 1995). These are also referred to as the 'essential elements' of any theory (Pearson and Vaughan, 1986).

Fawcett (1995) points out that every discipline has a metaparadigm; its purpose is to single out certain phenomena with which the discipline will deal. Most professions have a single metaparadigm from which numerous theories emerge – contemporary nursing appears to have reached this level of theoretical development.

During the 1970s and 1980s authors wrote extensively about the importance of the metaparadigm for nursing science. The argument was put forward that unless a conceptualisation included assumptions about nursing, health, person, and environment, it could not be considered to be a theory (Fitzpatrick and Whall 1996).

However, the complete four-element metaparadigm has its dissenters. For example, Stevens (1979) excludes 'environment', while Kim (1983) excludes 'health'. Others believe that 'nursing' should be omitted as a concept, maintaining that its inclusion is a redundancy of terms and that 'caring' should be included instead (Leininger, cited in Huch, 1995). However, to exclude nursing and include caring would mean that the resultant 'health, person, caring and environment' could well be perceived as a metaparadigm for medicine! The inclusion of nursing, however, may be seen as excluding midwifery and health visiting from the debate.

Since Fitzpatrick and Whall (1996) argue that the metaparadigm represents the foundation stones for nursing theories, one would expect each theorist to outline her (all the major nurse theorists are female) beliefs and assumptions regarding the person, to present an identification of the person's environment, to define her view of nursing and to discuss her views on health. Close examination of nursing theories shows that this is the case. Each theorist does conceptualise the four elements of the metaparadigm, but they tend to view them from different perspectives.

Therefore, how nursing, health, person and environment are described and defined varies greatly from theorist to theorist. So, while each one considers the metaparadigm, they may emphasise different aspects and see them in different relations to one another. Such a rich diversity of assumptions concerning the same factors will only serve to enrich our profession. Nightingale (1859), for instance, believed that nursing put the patient in the best condition for nature to act upon him. She placed great emphasis on the environment and the detrimental effect that poor environments had on people's health. Although she too dealt with each of the metaparadigm components, she focused specifically on the patient and the environment. Of the modern theorists, Martha Rogers (1980) was perhaps the most influential in continuing this emphasis on the importance of the environment.

To illustrate how some theorists have taken cognisance of the metaparadigm I have extracted the components from the works of Roper, Logan and Tierney (1990), Henderson (1966), Orem (1980) and Roy (1971).

Person/man

Definitions:

- Biological human beings with inseparable mind and body who share certain fundamental human needs (Henderson, 1966).
- An unfragmented whole who carries out or is assisted in carrying out those activities that contribute to the process of living (Roper, Logan and Tierney, 1990).
- A functional integrated whole with a motivation to achieve self-care (Orem, 1980).
- A bio-psycho-social being who presents as an integrated whole (Roy, 1971).

Nursing

Definitions:

- A profession whose focus is to help the client to prevent, solve, alleviate or cope with problems associated with the activities he or she carries out in order to live (Roper, Logan and Tierney, 1990).
- A profession that assists the person sick or well in the performance of those activities contributing to health or its recovery (or to a peaceful death) that he or she would perform unaided, given the necessary strength, will or knowledge (Henderson, 1966).
- A human service related to the clients' need and ability to undertake self-care and to help them sustain health, recover from disease and injury or cope with their effects (Orem, 1980).
- A socially valued service whose goal is to promote a positive adaptation to the stimuli and stresses encountered by the client (Roy, 1971).

Health

Definitions:

- The ability to function independently regarding fourteen activities of daily living (Henderson, 1966).

- The optimum level of independence in each activity of living which enables the individual to function at his/her maximum potential (Roper, Logan and Tierney, 1990).
- A state of wholeness or integrity of the individual, his parts and his modes of functioning (Orem, 1980).
- The adaptation of the person to stimuli on a continuous line between wellness and illness (Roy, 1971).

Environment

Definitions:

- That which may act in a positive or negative way upon the client (Henderson, 1966).
- Circumstances that may impinge upon the individual as he or she travels along the life-span and cause movement towards maximum dependence or maximum independence (Roper, Logan and Tierney, 1990).
- A sub-component of man, and with man forms an integrated system related to self-care (Orem, 1980).
- Both internal and external. From the environment people are subject to stresses (Roy, 1971).

Afaf Meleis, a highly influential author on theorising in nursing, uses the term 'domain' when referring to nursing's field of interest. Although it does not have the exact same components as the meta-paradigm, it has a similar meaning. She defines domain as 'the perspective and territory of a discipline' (Meleis, 1991: 12). She goes further than Fawcett and identifies seven concepts as central to the domain of nursing. These are: 'nursing client', 'transitions', 'interaction', 'nursing process', 'environment', 'nursing therapeutics' and 'health'.

To illustrate the relationship between these concepts Meleis (1991) believes that the nurse interacts (*interaction*) in a health/illness situation with a human being (*nursing client*) who is an integral part of his or her socio-cultural context (*environment*) and who is in some sort of transition or is anticipating a transition (*transition*); the nurse–patient interactions are organised around some purpose (*nursing process*), and the nurse uses some actions (*nursing therapeutics*) to enhance or facilitate health (*health*).

In her 1995 book, Fawcett ably addresses the criticisms levelled at her perception of the metaparadigm. She also appears to be coming closer to the ideas of Meleis in that she specifies that 'nursing' within her four-component metaparadigm does include nursing therapeutics, and 'person' does include groups and communities. In essence, therefore, both metaparadigm and domain are terms which may be used to identify those broad parameters of nursing.

Another global term often referred to in the literature is 'philosophy'. According to Silva (1986a) a philosophy is concerned with the nature of being, the nature of reality and the limits of knowledge. A philosophy is also perceived as 'a statement of beliefs and values about the world, a perspective on human beings and their world, and an approach to the development of knowledge' (Fawcett, 1992: 68). According to Salsberry (1994), a philosophy identifies what is believed to be the basic or central issues of a discipline. This latter definition illustrates that philosophy can have a similar meaning to metaparadigm or domain.

In this text Fawcett's definition of philosophy will be adopted. Therefore, while you may agree that the client is an essential part of the metaparadigm of nursing, two practitioners may have varying values and beliefs (*philosophy*) as to how they perceive the client: one may believe and value the client to be an independent self-caring individual while the other may believe and value the client to be a dependent person relying on the nurse to meet or help him or her meet basic needs.

Working terms

- Phenomenon
- Concept
- Construct
- Proposition

Phenomenon

A phenomenon (plural: phenomena) is a thing, event or activity that we perceive through our senses. I include in this the sixth sense

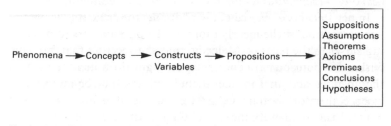

Figure 1.1 Representation of relationship between theoretical 'working terms'

of intuition or 'gut reaction'. You could say that phenomena represent the subject-matter of a discipline. It has been stated: 'when experience and sensory and intuitive data become coherent as a whole, and prior to any attachment of meaning, we have a phenomenon' (Meleis, 1991: 201). For instance, prior to surgery you may perceive a patient being restless in bed, you note that she is biting her nails, she is sighing, your hand on her brow tells you she is perspiring and clammy. As another example, you may note that elderly male patients on certain medications wander out of their bedroom between 3a.m. and 5a.m. and, when asked, do not know who they are or where they are. Other nurses you ask have also noted this behaviour. Prior to putting a name to either of these occurrences, you are noting a phenomenon. A phenomenon remains a phenomenon as long as no cognitive or inferential interpretation is attached to it.

Nurses must attend to those phenomena that are of central importance to nursing. We must guard against teaching and researching issues and basing our practice around phenomena which are of more interest to another discipline than they are to nursing. On occasions this happens, and authors like Meleis (1991) have urged nursing to get back to the substantive issues which hold relevance for nursing.

Concept

Meleis defines a concept as 'a label used to describe a phenomenon or a group of phenomena' (1991: 12). Therefore, when we put a name to a phenomenon we are identifying *concepts*. In the first example above you may label the phenomenon 'anxiety', while the second may be labelled 'early morning drug-related confusion'.

As a mental image, a concept is a view of reality tinted with the observer's perception, experience and philosophical bent. You should remember that the same phenomenon may be given a different conceptual label by two different nurses. Therefore, a concept is a tool and not a real entity – it merely facilitates observation of a real phenomenon. It refers to the properties of a phenomenon; the concept is not the phenomenon itself, rather it is a name one gives to a phenomenon. Concepts give meaning for filing purposes, enabling us to categorise, interpret and structure the phenomenon. Concepts are also the building blocks of theory, they convey the ideas within the theory. To Fawcett and Downs (1992) the concepts of a theory are its special vocabulary.

Construct

If the phenomena are very abstract and the resultant concept is not directly observable or measurable it is often referred to as a 'construct' (e.g., self-esteem). A construct is sometimes confused with the term 'concept'. But, according to Chinn and Kramer (1995), 'a construct is a type of highly complex concept whose reality base can only be inferred' (1995: 212). Therefore, if you could imagine a continuum of concepts from concrete (thermometer) to abstract (caring, compassion), constructs would be placed at the abstract end. You must remember that all constructs are concepts, but not all concepts are constructs.

Duldt and Griffin (1985) illustrate the continuum of abstraction of concepts in the following way. They identified a 'cow' as a very concrete conceptualisation and proceed through the following more abstract levels of conceptualisation: 'cow' – 'Bessie' – 'livestock' – 'farm asset' – 'asset' – 'wealth'. Two things are happening as the concepts become more abstract; more of the characteristics of the concept 'cow' are being omitted and the ability to directly observe and measure the concept is becoming more difficult.

Constructs may be made measurable by identifying 'variables'.

Powers and Knapp (1995: 166) define variable as 'an operationali-sation of a construct'. For example, if 'civil status' is perceived as a construct, it could be made measurable by breaking it into the vari-ables 'single' and 'widowed', 'divorced', 'married', etc.

Proposition

Different concepts, constructs and variables can be linked by state-ments of relationships. Such linking statements are called 'propositions'. Therefore, propositions are 'tentative statements about reality and its nature. They describe relationships between events, situations or actions' (Meleis, 1991: 205). The different types of proposition which go to make up theory will be discussed in greater depth in Chapter 3.

In the literature there are different types of propositional state-ment. These include:

● Assumption
● Supposition
● Premise
● Axiom
● Postulate
● Conclusion
● Hypothesis
● Theorem

An assumption is 'a notion that is widely accepted to be true' (George, 1985: 339). Assumptions are important parts of theories. In essence, they are taken-for-granted statements which may not have been proved or undergone empirical testing. 'Man is a bio-psycho-social being' is an assumption.

A supposition is another prepositional term which means the same as assumption. According to Chinn and Kramer (1995), supposi-tions are taken to be true for the sake of argument. We tend to accept the supposition that the environment is forever changing.

A premise is a relationship statement 'used in deductive logic as a basis for forming a conclusion' (Chinn and Kramer, 1995: 217).

This term will be explained further in Chapter 2, when deductive reasoning is discussed.

Axioms and postulates are similar to premises and form the major components within deductive logic. According to Marriner-Tomey (1994a: 4), an axiom is 'a statement from which other statements of a theory may be logically derived'.

A conclusion is also a propositional statement and is the end result of deductive reasoning. An example of deductive reasoning would be:

All staff on ward X are in the multidisciplinary team	1st premise (axiom/postulate)
Mary is a member of staff on ward X	2nd premise (axiom/postulate)
Therefore Mary is in the multidisciplinary team.	Conclusion (or theorem)

A hypothesis is also a proposition and has been defined by Chinn and Kramer (1995: 214) as 'a tentative statement which suggests some sort of relationship between two or more variables in a theory and can be tested through using research methods'. Therefore, hypotheses are statements of relationship between concepts stated in empirically testable terms.

A theorem is, again, the product of deductive reasoning. However, this term is most often encountered in mathematics and physics.

Like pieces in a puzzle, the foregoing terms form the infrastructure for theory development from practice. For example, suppose you continually observe that, after bowel surgery, male patients go to the toilet very frequently (phenomenon). You name this phenomenon 'post-op. urinary frequency' (concept). You develop a hunch that lower bowel surgery affects bladder capacity (proposition as a premiss). Over a two-month period you decide to test whether all males who undergo bowel surgery in your hospital state that they pass urine more frequently than normal (proposition as a hypothesis). By testing this hypothesis through a research study you may contribute to a theory which will provide new knowledge for the future care of such patients.

Middle terms

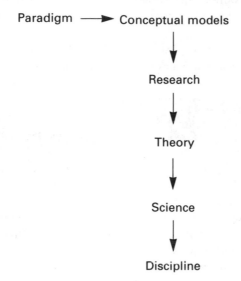

Figure 1.2 Representation of relationship between theoretical 'middle terms'

Under the global terms and made up of relationships between the working terms are what may be referred to as 'middle terms'. These include:

- Model
- Theory
- Paradigm
- Discipline
- Research
- Science

Theories and models have much in common: they tend to be composed of concepts and propositions that are systematically
constructed. Therefore, it is not surprising that there is much confusion and discussion among nurse scholars as to the difference
between these two terms. The arguments surrounding this confusion will be explored in detail below.

Model

Some of the simplest definitions of a model describe it as, 'a representation of reality' (McFarlane, 1986a), or a simplified way of
organising a complex phenomenon (Stockwell, 1985). Other
authors have elaborated on both these descriptions. Fawcett (1992)
states that a model is a set of concepts and the assumptions that
integrate them into a meaningful configuration. Rambo (1984)
believes that a model is a way of representing a situation in logical
terms in order to show the structure of the original idea or object.

A model train is a representation of a real train in the same way
that an architect's model office block represents the proposed building. It gives the viewer an indication of what the real thing is like. A
model of psychiatric nursing should provide a representation of
one way of viewing psychiatric nursing.

A model has also been described as 'a mental or diagrammatic
representation of care which is systematically constructed and
which assists practitioners in organising their thinking about what
they do, and in the transfer of their thinking into practice for the
benefit of the client and the profession' (McKenna, 1994b: 16).
Models, therefore, are conceptual tools or devices that can be used
by an individual to understand and place complex phenomena into
perspective. However, while conceptual models are supposed to
simplify complex issues, many nurses perceive nursing models as
doing the opposite – a common criticism of models being that they
overcomplicate nursing practice (McKenna, 1994b).

Models take various forms: Chapman (1985) used three dimensions to describe them. Those models that are presented in a
one-dimensional format take the form of verbal statements or
philosophical beliefs about phenomena. One-dimensional models
tend to be at a high level of abstraction. They cannot be taken

apart or explicitly observed, but they can be thought about and mentally manipulated.

Two-dimensional models include diagrams, drawings, graphs or pictures. Examples of such models include dress patterns, London Transport's underground plan, New York's bus routes and the diagrammatic representation of the amino acid chains. Most of the nursing models with which we are familiar began as one-dimensional conceptualisations in the theorists' minds and were later developed into two-dimensional formats.

Three-dimensional models are what Craig (1980) refers to as 'physical models'. These are scale models or structural replicas of things. In this form they may be minutely examined and manipulated. Examples of three-dimensional models include model toys, architectural scale models and anatomical models.

A one-dimensional model of the brain would be a verbal outline of its structure and function. A two-dimensional model would take the form of a diagram of the brain showing the various structures and how they relate to each other. This model will give you more information than the one-dimensional format. A three-dimensional model could take the form of a plastic teaching replica of the brain that could be taken apart and the internal structures removed and examined. This three-dimensional model gives you even more information about the structure and function of the brain than the previous one- and two-dimensional models.

All three classes of models bestow an enormous amount of information on those who use them. They tend to give you a simplified yet structured view of the particular phenomena under consideration. In this way you are able to understand the represented concepts and the relationship of those concepts to each other.

Models have been employed in all fields of scientific enquiry. Their function is the same regardless of discipline. They seek to clarify and elucidate. Mathematicians and engineers have used models for this purpose for thousands of years. In biology, Watson and Crick, who discovered the structure of DNA, postponed celebrations and publication until after they had constructed a two- and then a three-dimensional model of the helix.

Theory

The natural sciences of physics, astronomy, chemistry, biology, etc. have laws to explain how particular phenomena behave. Such laws enable scientists to predict with an absolute degree of certainty the results of a specific experiment. In nursing, because we are dealing with human beings and their complex realities, it is almost impossible to formulate laws. The best that can be done is to generate different types of theory to help us describe, explain, predict or control human behaviours.

One definition of theory, therefore, is as 'a set of concepts, definitions and propositions that project a systematic view of phenomena by designating specific interrelationships among concepts for the purpose of describing, explaining, predicting and/or controlling phenomena' (Chinn and Jacobs, 1987: 70). Duldt and Griffin (1985: 5) present a similar definition: 'a system of interrelated propositions which should enable phenomena to be described, explained, predicted and controlled'.

Because of the emphasis on prediction and control and the hierarchical nature of the definitions, these viewpoints appear to have their origins in empirical quantifiable science. In their most recent book, Chinn and Kramer have formulated a more qualitative definition with theory being perceived as 'a careful and rigorous structuring of ideas that project a tentative, purposeful and systematic view of phenomena' (1995: 220). Taking an equally broader definition, Barnum (1990: 16) offers the following: 'a theory is a statement that purports to account for or characterise some phenomenon'. This last definition is the least restrictive in defining theory while Duldt and Griffin's definition is probably the most restrictive. Therefore, what would be regarded as a theory by Barnum would not be regarded as such by Duldt and Griffin. This has implications for the differentiation between models and theories in nursing.

Nursing models or nursing theories?

Hildegard Peplau referred to her work as 'a set of concepts, a framework that can be applied to various kinds of nursing situations, but to call it a theory, I wouldn't' (cited in Suppe and Jacox, 1985: 243). Nevertheless, Stevens (1979) viewed Peplau's conceptualisation as a theory while Riehl and Roy (1980) called it a conceptual model. In a more recent book, Peplau (1995) does indeed refer to her work as a theory.

Similarly, Callista Roy's work on adaptation (1971) has been seen as a conceptual framework by Williams (1979), a grand theory by Kim (1983), an ideology by Beckstrand (1980) and as neither a model nor a theory by Webb (1986a). Dorothea Orem's work on self-care (1980) has also been the object of some semantic indistinctness. Suppe and Jacox (1985) believe Orem has constructed a conceptual framework, Johnson (1983) prefers to view it as a descriptive theory, Rosenbaum (1986) favours the title macro-theory, and the Nursing Theories Conference Group (George, 1985) recognises it as a conceptual model.

Notwithstanding these contradictory opinions, it is accepted by some authors that models are the most appropriate precursors of theory (Fawcett, 1995; Chinn and Kramer, 1995). This stance centres on their belief in the rigid criteria necessary for theory recognition and the inability of many 'nursing models' to meet them. Models are believed to lead to the identification of concepts and assumptions which, when tested by research, will ultimately lead to the formation of theory.

According to Fawcett (1995), models are more abstract than their theoretical counterparts. They present a more generalised and broader view of the phenomena under study. Theories, on the other hand, are more specific and precise, containing more clearly defined concepts with a narrower focus. The difference, therefore, is one of abstraction, explication and application. I will refer to this argument as Position A (see Figure 1.3).

Figure 1.3 would appear to clear up any confusion between models and theories. However, taking a different stance from that of Jacqueline Fawcett (1995), a group of metatheorists, ably represented by Afaf Meleis (1995) and Barbara Stevens-Barnum (1994), argue that it matters little what we call these things. They believe that much time has been wasted debating the differences between models and theories. Rather, time would be better spent evaluating the effects of these on client care. Other disciplines are not caught

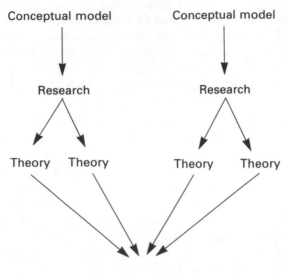

Figure 1.3   The model–theory debate – Position A

up in semantic tangles. For instance, Freud's (1949) work was not based on rigorous research, yet we refer to it as Freudian theory not Freudian model. Meleis wonders why nurses have to denigrate their theoretical work to such an extent that it does not merit the title theory. 'These differences are tentative at best and hair-splitting, unclear, and confusing at worst' (Meleis, 1991: 16).

Meleis and Stevens-Barnum base their arguments on their desire to concentrate on content and not on labels. They assert that theory exists at different stages of development, from the most primitive to the most sophisticated form and, therefore, even the simplest conceptualisation is a theory. They assert that models are theories but at a more abstract level than those theories developed through research. It mainly depends on the number of phenomena the theory addresses.

The sociologist Merton (1968) identified three categories of theory: grand theory, middle-range theory and narrow-range theory (practice theories). Grand theory is highly abstract and is broad in scope. Middle-range theory is more focused and is normally the end product of a research study. Narrow-range theory is even more specific and while also being based upon research findings, it guides specific actions in the achievement of desirable goals. More will be said about these categorisations in later chapters.

Using such categorisation, Roy's (1971) work would be designated a grand theory. However, it is possible to study the 'adaptation modes' component of Roy's work and, as a result of the research, produce a mid-range 'self-concept' theory. It may also be possible to examine the self-concept mode and identify a narrow-range theory concerning promoting adaptation within the self-concept mode of patients in British intensive care units. The former may be referred to as grand (or broad) theories, while the latter are referred to as middle-range or practice theories, respectively. This argument will be known as Position B (see Figure 1.4).

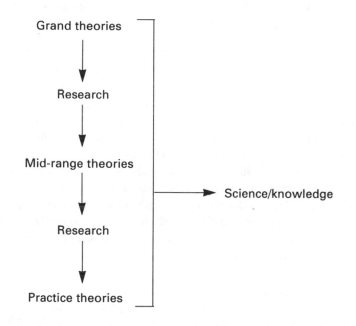

Figure 1.4 The theory–model debate – Position B

Both Position A and Position B can be supported by referring to various literature. I would urge the reader to view both approaches as worthy of consideration: the choice of whether you use the term 'model' or 'theory' is very much a personal matter. Personally, I prefer the term 'grand theory' instead of 'model'. The basis for this preference lies with Meleis's call for professionals to move towards a common language and to concentrate on substance (content), not on circular debates concerning structure (terminology). While accepting the existence of Merton's (1968) three categorisations of theory, when theories are mentioned in the remainder of this book, I will be referring to grand theories (models) unless otherwise specified.

Paradigm

The word 'paradigm' derives from the Greek word *paradeigma*, meaning pattern. Modern usage of the term in theoretical thinking originated with Thomas Kuhn's work in 1962 (see Chapter 2 of this volume). Fawcett (1992: 66) maintains that a paradigm represents 'global ideas about the individuals, groups, situations and events of interest to a discipline'. In the literature, paradigms are often seen as synonymous with the term 'model' (see Robinson, 1994: 13; Powers and Knapp, 1995: 118; Moody, 1990: 35; Peplau, 1987: 22; Kuhn, 1970: 174). However, others view paradigms as being much broader than models, representing a world view (Stevens-Barnum, 1994). Like all theoretical terms, paradigm has had many different definitions. Kuhn himself appeared confused when he used the term in twenty-one different ways (Masterman, 1970).

There are four main paradigms which may be used for the classification of nursing theories. The paradigms have been identified as: 'systems', 'interactional', and 'developmental' (Barnum-Stevens, 1994). Some nursing theories also have a large behavioural basis, and so the 'behavioural' paradigm has been included as a fourth category (Grahame, 1987).

Systems paradigm

Theories within this paradigm are largely based upon the 'general systems' paradigm as put forward by Von Bertalanffy (1951). Put simply, a system is a collection of parts that function as a whole entity for a particular purpose. Therefore, the parts within a particular system are interrelated. These interrelationships may form 'subsystems' within the parent system. Similarly, the system itself may form part of an overall 'suprasystem'. If the system has permeable boundaries it is called an 'open system'. In those nursing theories that have their roots within the system paradigm, the client is often referred to as an 'open system'.

Within this paradigm every event and occurrence can be perceived as a system. You may perceive a patient as a system made up of subsystems (respiratory system, cardiac system, etc.). He or she may live within a larger suprasystem (e.g., family, class grouping). This system interacts openly with other systems and has permeable boundaries because there are inputs into the system (knowledge, food, water, etc.) and outputs (waste, speech, perspiration, etc.).

You may also have identified a hospital ward as a system that contains beds and clients (subsystems) and is part of a larger unit or hospital (suprasystem). These systems are 'open systems' because people or matter pass from suprasystem to system and vice versa. The work of Roy (1971), Neuman (Neuman and Young, 1972) and Johnson (1959) has been recognised as having its basis within the systems paradigm.

Interactional paradigm

Interactional theories have their origin in the symbolic interactionist paradigm (Blumer, 1969). This paradigm emphasises the relationships between people and the roles they play in society. Nursing activities are perceived as interactional processes between practitioners and clients.

Supporters of the interaction paradigm can reasonably explain all human activities as interactions. For example, when nurses assess a client there is an interaction taking place leading to a transaction of information. Furthermore, the interaction, and the results of it, may be decided by the various roles the practitioners and the clients play. The nurses react to the clients' interaction and vice versa, and nurses may alter their own interactional processes as a result of reactions from the clients. Among the better-known theories which have their basis within this paradigm are those of Riehl (1974), Orlando (1961) and King (1968).

Developmental paradigm

The developmental paradigm originated from the work of Freud (1949) and Sullivan (1953). The central themes are growth, development, maturation and change. Within this paradigm, it is argued that human beings are constantly developing whether this be physiologically, socially, cognitively, psychologically or spiritually. Development is seen as an ongoing process in which the person must pass through various stages. The nurse's role is to encourage positive development and to break down or discourage the formation of barriers to natural development.

Within this paradigm, nurses are perceived as encouraging growth and development much as a gardener would do with plants. The client may have had an amputation and have to live with a new disability. Initially, care will be required if these clients are to learn new attitudes, knowledge and skills in order to mature in the new situation in which they find themselves. Hopefully, their care will reach a point where they will no longer require the support and presence of the nurse because they will have changed to a higher level of growth within the limits of the disability. The works of Peplau (1952), Travelbee (1966) and Newman (1979) are often perceived as having their foundations in the developmental paradigm.

Behavioural paradigm

The behavioural paradigm owes much to the theoretical formulations of Abraham Maslow (1954) concerning motivation. Because of this, the theories which emanate from it are often referred to as 'human needs' theories' (Webb, 1986b). The behavioural paradigm assumes that individuals normally exist and survive by meeting their own needs.

Nurses and midwives may perceive humans as having certain basic (e.g., food) and advanced (support) needs. On occasions, clients may be unable to meet these needs and staff may either assist them or teach them how to meet the needs in other ways or involve family members in meeting the person's needs. The works of Henderson (1966), Roper, Logan and Tierney (1990), Orem (1980), Minshull, Ross and Turner (1986) and Wiedenbach (1964) appear to have been influenced by the behavioural paradigm.

It would be a mistake to view these paradigms as being mutually exclusive. There is much overlap between and a degree of confusion among the various proponents. However, each one does present a view of how nurses can perceive people, health, nursing and environment. Further, because there are no rigid criteria available to allocate theories into these paradigmatic classifications, disagreements have occurred between authors over to which grouping a particular theory belongs. For instance, Orem's work has been seen as having its basis in the systems paradigm by Suppe and Jacox (1985), in the interactional paradigm by Greaves (1984), in the developmental paradigm by McFarlane (1986a) and in the behavioural paradigm by Chapman (1985). Notwithstanding these disagreements, this paradigmatic method of development and classification has been considered a valid one for nursing theories.

Yet another definition of a paradigm describes it as 'an action plan that describes the work to be done in a discipline and frames an orientation within which the work will be accomplished' (Powers and Knapp, 1995: 118). This definition intimates that paradigms also influence the research being carried out by a discipline and the methods of enquiry used.

Discipline

Nursing as a discipline is seen as being different from nursing as a science. The distinction is not just semantic. The following citation should indicate the difference:

> A discipline is characterised by a unique perspective, a distinct way of viewing all phenomena, which ultimately defines the limits and nature of its inquiry. Nursing as a discipline is broader than nursing as a science. Its uniqueness stems from its perspective rather than the focus of enquiry or methods of enquiry.
>
> (Donaldson and Crowley, 1978: 114)

Research

Research may be defined as 'a systematic process of enquiry which utilises a variety of methodological approaches to investigate the questions and concepts of interest in nursing' (Hinshaw, 1989: 163). Research aims to increase the sum total of our knowledge through systematic enquiry. This view of research is broad and covers both qualitative and quantitative research approaches. In contrast, Kerlinger (1986: 10) defines research as 'a systematic, controlled, empirical and critical investigation of natural phenomena guided by theory and hypotheses about the presumed relations among such phenomena'. This view of research is reminiscent of those who favour a narrow empirical approach to theory generation and testing.

Science

While I will be returning to different views of science in later chapters, a definition here will show how it fits with the other terms dealt with in this chapter. Meleis (1991: 11) states that science is 'a unified body of knowledge about phenomena that is supported by agreed upon evidence'. Put more simply, Powers and Knapp (1995) view science as an activity that combines research and theory: therefore, Science = Research + Theory.

In many instances when nurses talk of science it is interpreted as cold, objective, controlled and detached. However, there is also 'human science', the definition of which may be more acceptable to nursing: 'science is nothing else than the search to discover unity in the wild variety of nature or . . . in the variety of our experiences' (Bronowski, 1965: 16). Therefore, science is an organised way of viewing the world in which we live. It is about understanding and explanation, and not just control. This definition sets the tone for this book, which is built on the notion that there are various methods and approaches to the development, application and evaluation of knowledge in nursing.

In particular 'nursing science' has been defined by Stevenson and Woods (1985: 7) as a domain of knowledge concerned with the adaptation of individuals and groups to actual and potential health problems, the environments that influence health in humans, and the therapeutic interventions that promote health and affect the consequences of illness.

In essence, science is how we view the world; research is the tool of science and theory is the product. So the linkage between theory and research will give us science, and science is the body of knowledge that determines whether a group of people working towards a common goal represent a discipline.

Summary

This chapter has focused upon theoretical terms with which at this stage you may be unfamiliar. I have arbitrarily divided these terms into global, working and middle terms. Global terms relate to a very broad world view concerning the knowledge base of professions. Working terms are those elements, such as concepts and propositions, that come together to form middle terms such as theories and models. These are the building blocks of the knowledge base for any discipline.

It has to be stated that the terminology surrounding theory and the development of knowledge generally is complex, and it would not be unusual for you to come across definitions which differ in perspective from those given above. However, while it would be possible to write a textbook on theoretical terminology alone, you should be aware of the lack of agreement on terms and that we should continually search for consensus. I will be referring to these terms throughout this book and, as a result, they should, I hope, become more 'user-friendly' as you continue reading.

Chapter 2
Ways of knowing

This chapter will introduce you to the different ways of knowing and how these are applied to nursing. This will form the philosophical background to later chapters which deal specifically with the generation, selection, application and testing of nursing theory.

It would be a useful starting-point if we looked at definitions of knowing and of knowledge. According to Chinn and Kramer (1995) *knowing* refers to the individual human processes of experiencing and comprehending the self and the world in ways that can be brought to some level of conscious awareness. Therefore, because it alters with experience, knowing is seldom static. But not all knowing can be covered by Chinn and Kramer's definition.

Buber (1962) extracts the following from the Talmud:

> the child in the womb of his mother looks from one end of the world to the other and knows all the teaching, but the instant he comes in contact with the air of earth an angel strikes him on the mouth and he forgets everything.
>
> (cited in Levine, 1994)

But perhaps everything is not forgotten; people are born with what may be termed 'instinctive knowing', i.e., the instincts of survival such as those of blinking and swallowing, and the physiological flight–fright response to threats, for example.

Knowledge, in contrast, is defined as knowing that can be shared or communicated with others (Chinn and Kramer, 1995). Therefore, knowledge may be communicated and become part of other people's repertoire of knowing. You may be aware that, before they get their licence, trainee taxi drivers in London must obtain 'the knowledge'. This represents knowledge of the city and is communicated to trainees through maps, the written word and their own experience of travelling the streets. In nursing too, we obtain knowledge through experience and the written word. We also use maps in the form of theories that tell us where we are, or should be, going (Clark, 1986).

Philosophies of knowledge

There are three dominant philosophical views on how knowledge develops.

- Rationalism
- Empiricism
- Historicism

Each of these has had an impact on the ways in which nurses justify why they know what they know.

Rationalism

Rationalism comes from the Latin word for 'reason'. It is a philosophy of science which emphasises the role that reason has to play in the development of knowledge and the discovery of truth. It is founded on the idea that scholars, without access to data obtained through the senses, can generate theory through mental reasoning. They do this by formulating hypotheses and propositions through 'armchair theorising' and then setting up an experiment to see if the theory can be corroborated in the real world. This can be described as the 'theory-then-research' approach (Reynolds, 1971). Because the theory comes first, this approach to knowledge development can also be called deductive or a priori reasoning. The end result may be an accepted theory, a refuted theory, a modified theory or a call for further testing of the theory. Since Einstein's theory of relativity was formed many years before the methods were available to test it, it is perhaps the best-known example of knowledge development through rationalism.

Rationalism as an approach to scientific knowledge development can be traced to René Descartes (1596–1650), the seventeenth-century French philosopher. Descartes, who spent most of his adult life in Holland, influenced the Dutch philosopher Baruch Spinoza, who also became a leading rationalist.

In his book *Meditations on First Philosophy* (1641) Descartes realised that to arrive at new knowledge you must cast doubt on former opinions and experiences. When we do this we can then build truth and knowledge from first foundations.

Descartes admitted that most of what we believe to be real is learned through the senses, yet the senses can play tricks on us. For example, we may think something looks cold but, when we touch it, it is warm, or we may be deceived into believing that a branch touching a window is someone knocking. Accepting this as a basis, he asks us to imagine that an evil genie is consistently fooling us by sending false sensory information and that, as a result, what we perceive through the senses does not exist at all!

When Descartes took this as his basis he came to the conclusion that all that he previously held to be true and to exist was now in doubt. He also began to doubt his own existence; however, he reasoned that he must exist or he would not be doubting everything in the first place. He must exist, he reasoned, as a mind that thinks and reasons. At this stage Descartes wrote the famous words 'Cogito, ergo sum' (I think, therefore I am).

Descartes was a devout Catholic and reasoned that God created two classes of substance that make up the whole of reality. One class was thinking substances, or minds, and the other was extended substances, or bodies. This mind–matter split, called 'Cartesian dualism', is based on the assumption that we are rational individuals with rational minds and that our minds are divorced from our bodies and other matter. He held that, by means of reason alone, knowledge and certain universal, self-evident truths could be discovered, from which the sciences could be derived deductively.

Descartes' method of reasoning did not always come up with the truth as we know it today. He believed that the blood was made up in part of fluid, which he called 'animal spirits'. The animal spirits, he believed, came into contact with thinking substances in the brain and flowed out along the channels of the nerves to animate the muscles and other parts of the body.

None the less, rationalism as a philosophy of science was very influential. The perception within the medical model that a person is made of anatomical parts and physiological systems can be traced back to the mind–body split as propounded by Descartes.

When nurses assess patients objectively from a physical and pathological perspective while ignoring their emotions and feelings they are practising Descartesian dualism.

In addition, the deductive reasoning approach as expounded by Descartes became a keystone of modern scientific enquiry. Carl Popper (1965), a leading philosopher of science, was influenced by Descartes. He argued that the way to true knowledge was by conjecture (developing theory through reason) and refutation (testing the theory through rigorous research).

Empiricism

Empiricism is a philosophy of science which believes that knowledge is derived entirely from sensory experience. In other words, if something cannot be perceived through the five senses, it does not exist. In contrast to rationalism, it denies the possibility of spontaneous ideas or a priori reasoning as a precursor to scientific knowledge. Empiricism can be described as the 'research-then-theory' approach (Reynolds, 1971). In essence, theorists experience a phenomenon through their senses and they identify concepts and propositions that attempt to explain what they perceive. These propositions may go to form the basis of hypotheses which can be tested through experimental research. The end result is knowledge in the form of theory. Because the theory comes last, this approach to knowledge development can also be called inductive or a posteriori reasoning.

The origin of empiricism can be traced to the English philosophers of the seventeenth, eighteenth and nineteenth centuries. Of these, John Locke (1632–1704) was the first to put forward empiricist principles, although his fellow countryman, Francis Bacon (1561–1626), had anticipated some of empiricism's characteristic conclusions. Bacon argued that men's (*sic*) minds made hasty generalisations which prevented the attainment of knowledge. Most of these generalisations were based upon insufficient examination of the phenomena. Knowledge through reasoning was seen by Bacon as an invention of the imagination without any intellectual value.

Over a century later, the French philosopher Auguste Comte (1798–1857), who also founded sociology as a discipline, gave empiricism a new twist. Comte was influenced by the teachings of Descartes (Parker, 1991) and Locke. He was a politically aware, anti-establishment figure who identified science as being the key to political reconstruction. In his six-volume work, *Course of Positive Philosophy* (1830–42), he identified a three-state law of scientific development as shown in Box 2.1:

Box 2.1 Comte's three states of scientific development

The theological or fictitious state: This state is indicative of science before the twelfth century, where most events were explained by the will of God. Politically at this time power was represented by the divine right of kings.

The metaphysical or abstract state: This state is indicative of science in the Middle Ages, where events were explained by appealing to abstract philosophy. The political base at this time equated with the democratic social contract and the equality of individuals.

The scientific or positive state: Comte referred to this as the 'positive state' in order to differentiate it from the negative thinking of the previous two states. Here, events are explained by rigorous scientific observation. The political power is placed in the hands of a scientific elite where scientific methods would be used to solve human problems and improve social conditions.

The positivist approach to science as perceived by Comte became very influential and many scientists argued that positivism was the only true source of knowledge. In essence, the doctrine involved the following logic: our minds interpret the world through our senses, and because the world is subject to the laws of science, events outside the mind can be observed, described, explained and predicted. Therefore, in order to make sense of the outside world all we have to do is study it empirically and undertake experiments to test hypotheses that are formulated from observing this natural world.

Proponents of positivism believed that knowledge and objective truth existed and that the goal of science was to go out and discover it.

Comte also identified a hierarchy of six sciences which had been founded on systematic observation (astronomy, biology, chemistry, mathematics, physics and sociology). These form the 'gold standard' against which other disciplines would be judged. In contrast, subjective approaches to knowledge development were not perceived as meaningful pursuits and so reflection and intuition as a basis for knowledge development was shunned and denigrated by positivists.

Comte, who eventually succumbed to mental illness, wished to turn his beliefs into a religion. As a result, many erstwhile likeminded positivists began to move away from his teaching. At the turn of the century a group of philosophers calling themselves the 'Vienna Circle' (e.g., Schlick, Wittgenstein) left behind Comte's ideas of personal experience as the basis for true knowledge and coined the term 'logical positivism'. This placed a stronger emphasis on the importance of induction and scientific verification (Emden, 1991).

For most of the twentieth century 'respected' scientists adopted the logical positivist view of science. However, the philosophical force behind logical positivism dissipated just prior to the Second World War, when most of its supporters had left Nazi Germany and Austria. Almost sixty years later, in the latter part of the twentieth century, it is seen as a spent force in scientific enquiry.

It is interesting that Whall (1989), as a result of studying nursing practice guides for the years 1950–70, found little evidence of the effect of positivism on nursing practice. She questioned Suppe and Jacox's (1985) assertion that nursing theory was strongly influenced by positivism. How could positivism influence theory but not practice? As if to answer this question Meleis (1991) was unable to uncover much evidence that positivistic thought had any effect on the development of nursing theory. Gortner (1993) strongly supports this viewpoint and urges nurses to resist further discussions on the long-extinct logical positivist influences.

Karl Popper (1965), initially a supporter of the Vienna Circle, began to reject induction as a scientific approach and replaced verification by the principle of falsification. In other words, theories should not be tested to see if they can be supported; rather, they should be tested to see if they can be falsified. If you test a theory nineteen times and it holds true nineteen times it may not hold true on the twentieth occasion. We can learn much more from the twentieth test than from the previous nineteen. For example, imagine theory as a paper boat which you push out into a pond. If it floats on nineteen occasions but sinks on the twentieth, you realise that there was something wrong with its construction or with the conditions in which it was used. Popper also questioned the logical positivists' desire to reject subjectivity as a way of knowing. He admitted that there was a place for intuition and imagination when one is using scientific empiricism.

This was not the first time that empiricism had been questioned. Immanuel Kant (1724–1804), the German philosopher, had attempted a compromise between empiricism and rationalism (Kant, trans. 1953). He restricted knowledge to the domain of experience, thus agreeing with the empiricists, but he attributed to the mind a function in incorporating sensations into the structure of experience, thus favouring reasoning.

Today, thanks to philosophers like Popper, logical positivism has been replaced by post-positivist empiricism, a much milder form of positivism. Gortner (1993) supports the use of this form of empiricism in the development of nursing science and sees as unfortunate the fact that it is still being tarnished in the literature through being confused with logical positivism. Modern empiricists accept the shortcomings of verification; they focus on observable phenomena and on research findings that can be confirmed and collaborated. They recognise that the world is complex and that some behaviours and events can be reduced for study purposes while others cannot (Gortner, 1993). Empiricism is still highly regarded as a scientific approach in the physical sciences of biology, physics and chemistry. Furthermore, many of the experiments, quasi-experiments and randomised controlled trials carried out within medicine and nursing show clear elements of this empiricism. Referring to nursing theories, Gortner (1993: 481) argues that Roy's (1989) theoretical thinking 'reflects clearly the thinking of an empiricist scholar'.

Historicism

There are many aspects of knowledge and truth that are subjective and to which the true rationalist or empirical principles could not apply. The philosophy of science best suited to this perspective is historicism. Historicism recognises that we are all influenced by our history and the experiences, values and beliefs we have thereby acquired. Because we construct our own realities and interpret events based upon our personal construction of the world, this view of science may also be referred to as the 'interpretative-constructionist' approach.

Readers may accept that knowledge is in the eye of the beholder. For instance, several nurses may observe the same clinical phenomenon, yet reflection and intuition may lead them to understand and interpret it differently. Furthermore, they each may have a personal or internationally accepted theory which structures what they perceive. Such 'theoretical baggage' influences both what is experienced and how we attempt to understand it. One nurse's interpretation of a clinical phenomenon may be based upon sociological theory while another, viewing the same situation, may be using organisational theory or counselling theory. So, to different people, reality (and knowledge of that reality) is a personal and therefore a variable thing, being the product of individual reflection, perception, perspective and purpose rather than being static and objective.

Realising this, philosophers such as Kuhn (1970), Toulmin (1972) and Feyerabend (1975) challenged the positivist view and stressed the importance of history and previous knowledge in the development of science. They dismissed the idea of objective truths. Rather, they argued that knowledge development is dynamic and so there are no final and permanent truths.

Thomas Kuhn saw science as a social activity. In 1962 he stated that science progressed through a series of revolutionary steps. Between each revolution there is a period of 'normal science', where a particular paradigm reigns supreme and scholars accept it as a basis for knowledge and truth. However, at some stage this paradigm is questioned because it fails to deal adequately with some new phenomenon. As more evidence accumulates to show that it has outlived its usefulness a 'paradigm shift' occurs through another revolution. According to Kuhn, paradigm shifts are not cumulative and the new paradigm is not built on the previous paradigm. The new paradigm becomes the focus for a new period of normal science.

Examples of this way of viewing knowledge would include the pre-Galileo view of the sun orbiting the earth or the beliefs held as true by the 'flat earth' society or the focus on community care as opposed to institutional care for those with mental health problems. Paradigm shifts occurred because these paradigms (world views) were not able to explain new experiences or solve new problems. These views of Kuhn's did much to undermine the empirical/positivist view of science.

Larry Laudan (1977) challenged Kuhn's (1970) view that knowledge development was a revolutionary process. Rather, he believed that knowledge was developed in an evolutionary way, with new knowing being influenced by previous knowing. This evolutionary approach of Laudan is an attractive one for nurses because it recognises a pluralistic approach to knowledge development and application. After all, the problems facing nursing are forever changing and staff must select the theory and paradigm best suited to solving the problems of relevance. Therefore, there can seldom be a consistent way of viewing nursing's reality because it is forever changing and giving rise to new problems.

However, Afaf Meleis (1991) argued that the revolutionary and evolutionary approaches are too simplistic on their own to explain nursing's experience of knowledge development. She coined the term 'convolutionary' to explain how nursing knowledge has developed. She maintains that nursing as a discipline has progressed not through evolution or revolution but through a convolutionary series of peaks, troughs, detours, backward steps and crises.

Further, there has been an increasing realisation in nursing that knowledge and knowing are not all about detached facts, objective data and people being understood by reducing them to a number of parts. Rather, people are more than the sum of their parts. To illustrate this, we can take the example of a birthday cake with a message 'Happy Birthday Mary' written on it. When we cut the cake into slices we lose the meaning of the message and we cannot understand it merely from viewing a slice of the cake. Putting the slices back together will still not give us the essence of the occasion. The cake, and the emotional meaning attached to it, is more than just the sum of the slices.

This leads us away from rationalism and positivism and to other ways of knowing. For instance, Husserl (1859–1938) argued that, because of its refusal to deal with anything other than observable entities and objective reality, positivism was not capable of dealing with human experience. He maintained that one way to truth was to consider the essences of things, and the best way of noting the essence of a thing was to see what meaning the mind has for that thing (Husserl, trans. 1962).

Phenomenology is the study of the meaning of phenomena to a particular individual, a way of understanding people from the way things appear to them (George, 1995). The task of phenomenology is to discover what 'life experiences' are like for people. The essence of people's existence is the experience and meanings they have in the world in which they live. Understanding this 'lived experience' requires the use of reflection, which is the basis of phenomenology. Husserl also recommended that phenomenologists 'bracket existence'. This means that they should suspend previous views and influences when they are exploring the essence of an occurrence or event. According to Powers and Knapp (1995), phenomenologists do not separate the act of perception from that being perceived. The perceived world is the real world. This differs significantly from the positivist approach of separating the observer (the researcher/theorist) from the observed (phenomena/subjects). Martin Heidegger, a student of Husserl, argued that, as a way of generating knowledge, phenomenology should make manifest what is hidden in everyday taken-for-granted experience. He disagreed with Husserl's (trans. 1962) idea that an observer can 'bracket existence'. Rather, he argued that prior experiences and influences may be used positively in a phenomenological study.

Hermeneutics, a branch of phenomenology much influenced by Heidegger, is based upon the idea that all texts and human activities are filled with meaning and should be subject to rigorous interpretations on the basis of these intrinsic meanings. Therefore, to know, within hermeneutics, is to understand through interpretation. Once more the hard science is being softened to take account of meaning and perception rather than detached quantification.

Gortner (1993) criticises the hermeneutic approach because it does not allow realism and explanations that are not subjective. It does not recognise the building of theory outside that of the person and their lived experience. In this regard, Gortner argues, it is no better than logical positivism and may also become extinct by virtue of these constraints.

Contemporaneous to the Vienna Circle, a group of philosophers existed who were referred to as the Frankfurt School. The School grew up around the work of Max Horkheimer and was very much anti-positivist in its teachings. While agreeing that the positivistic focus on sense experiences was fine for the natural sciences, the Frankfurt School viewed this as an erroneous way of viewing knowledge development in the social sciences. The Frankfurt scholars were firm exponents of the critical science approach.

Critical science is also a variant of phenomenology, but it goes beyond phenomenology in stressing that meanings should not be merely elicited but should be open to criticism. According to Powers and Knapp (1995), critical science is based on the belief that humans are typically dominated by social conditions that they can neither understand nor control, and that, when they become enlightened about the ideologies that oppress and constrain them, they become free and empowered. This is an attractive approach for those nurses who wish to leave behind subservience to the male-dominated medical model. It has given rise to feminist research methodologies and as such may be perceived as a science of freedom. There are three major concepts within critical theory, as shown in Box 2.2.

Therefore, critical theory assumes that all research and theory are socio-political constructions; that human societies are by their nature oppressive; and that all views and interpretations of the world are open to criticism. This focus on education, enlightenment, emancipation, empowerment, critique and change is an attractive perspective to many nurses and the increase in the number of action research studies in nursing in recent years supports this point.

> **Box 2.2 Three major concepts of critical theory**
>
> *Enlightenment:* knowledge of self in relation to the world and education of the oppressed in terms of their potential capacity to bring about change;
>
> *Empowerment:* social transformation through some form of educative process;
>
> *Emancipation:* a state of reflective clarity where people have a sense of themselves and can freely and collectively determine the directions they should take in life.
>
> (Emden, 1991)

Ways of knowing in nursing

The foregoing section on how different philosophies of science have influenced the way knowledge is obtained and perceived will now be applied to nursing. Most nurses have long accepted that people undergoing care deserve interventions which are based on sound knowledge. Florence Nightingale (1859) in the mid-nineteenth century, argued that nurses require a body of knowledge that is distinct from that of physicians. Nightingale was acutely aware of the positivist view of science and she would have been a proponent of that philosophy. She excelled in statistical analysis of extant data and the research approaches she used in studying conditions in the British army tended to favour a positivist methodology.

Nightingale did explicitly state propositions for nursing; for instance, she wrote about the positive relationship between an individual's health (abstract concept) and fresh air (abstract concept). As a result of this and similar conceptualising, she was probably the first nurse theorist. Fifty years after her death, other nurse theorists became committed to the same principle of developing an organised body of nursing knowledge for the purpose of guiding practice. One such theorist, Dorothy Johnson (1959: 291), asserted that 'no profession can long exist without making explicit its theoretical basis for practice so that this knowledge can be communicated, tested and expanded'. She further argued that society will only give nurses the authority and responsibility for practice if there is proof that they possess the knowledge required to do the job.

If nursing does not have a distinct body of knowledge, then we must have a distinct way of looking at a borrowed body of knowledge. If we have neither, we could ask, what is the basis for our existence as a discipline? After all, one of the hallmarks of a profession is that it possesses a body of knowledge pertaining to its craft.

In her later writings, Johnson (1968) argued that knowledge does not belong to any one group or discipline. She stated that, even if one discipline discovers or creates knowledge, this in itself does not confer the right of ownership. Therefore, a body of knowledge formulated within a specific discipline belongs to the world at large and, as a result, there is no nursing knowledge, merely knowledge that nurses use in a particular way. I will be returning to this theme of borrowed versus home-grown theory in Chapter 5.

'Know how' versus 'know that' knowledge

It is possible to differentiate nursing into what Schon (1987) would call the 'high hard ground' world of academia and the 'swampy lowlands' of practice. Knowledge in the former is more theoretic and abstract, while knowledge in the latter is continually altering in complexity, existing in a state of instability and uncertainty. Knowledge in the 'swamp' is also full of value conflicts (Meave, 1994).

These two types of knowledge had previously been described by Rhyl (1963) as 'know how knowledge' and 'know that knowledge'. The former is skills-based and involves knowing how to do something. This may include how to word-process an assignment or how to drive a car. You may know how to do these tasks without knowing either how a computer is programmed or the mechanical theory of the internal combustion engine. In nursing, much of 'know how knowledge' is based on intuition and is perceived as our 'art' and therefore has its roots in the historicism philosophy of science. In contrast, 'know that knowledge' has its basis in theory and empirical research and is often perceived as our 'science'. The value system underlying 'know that knowledge' is aligned to the philosophy of empiricism.

It is well documented that there is a rift between the 'know how knowledge' of clinical practice and the 'know that knowledge' taught in the classroom (Chambers, 1995). Because of the heavy influence of empiricism, the former is often perceived as less important than the latter. Practitioners are continually being urged to implement research findings with the hidden assumption that what they are doing in practice (know how knowledge) is incorrect and perhaps even wasteful and detrimental to clients. Meave (1994: 10) states that the elite in nursing occupy the 'high hard ground' and possess a great deal of knowledge about 'that'. The working class of nurses populate the 'swamp' and possess a great deal of knowledge about 'how'. Actual practice is different from theories of practice, because each reality is generated from different people living in different worlds.

There is, however, an increasing realisation of the value of 'know how knowing'. But, as argued by Chinn and Kramer (1995), knowing only becomes knowledge when it is communicated to others in word or deed, and 'know how knowing' cannot always be fully expressed. Experienced practitioners know intuitively what is good practice but they often have difficulty explaining exactly what they do. It is also possible that 'experienced' patients also know what constitutes good practice but they too have difficulty explaining what it is.

A study by Patricia Benner (1983) using a phenomenological approach identified how novices in nursing need quite rigid rules, procedures and guidelines to enable them to feel secure within clinical situations. Expert nurses, on the other hand, often find such rules an unnecessary encumbrance and mostly practise intuitively. It is particularly interesting that, in many instances, these expert nurses are unable to explain precisely why or how they know certain things.

Previously, Polanyi (1958) identified this phenomenon and called it 'tacit knowing' to distinguish it from 'explicit knowing'. Slevin (1995) defines tacit knowledge as a high degree of capacity to function with expertise without having to think, explain or problem-solve, indeed often being unable to explain why it is 'just known' that something is right in a particular situation. This definition places tacit knowing firmly within the category of 'know how knowledge'.

Miller (1989) identified the differences between 'know that' and 'know how' knowledge, as shown in Table 2.1.

Table 2.1 'Know how' versus 'know that' knowledge

Know how knowledge	Know that knowledge
Often inarticulate conceptualisations communicated by word of mouth or role-modelling	Articulated conceptualisations communicated as theories (e.g., Orem, Roy, Rogers, Neuman)
Based on personal experience	Based on invented or discovered reality
For the purpose of delivering care	For the purpose of describing, explaining, predicting, or prescribing care

If theory was based upon 'know how knowledge' it might be easier for practitioners to accept it as being appropriate for their practice. One way of achieving this is to use a phenomenological approach to knowledge development. As alluded to above, phenomenology encourages the generation of theoretical knowledge through exploring the meaning and experience of, among other things, 'know how' practice. This can lead to the generation of new theories having their foundations in the 'know how' knowledge of practitioners.

Practitioners could also bridge the theory–practice gap by being encouraged and supported to apply research and theory to their practice. In this way, 'know how' knowledge would be the conduit for putting 'know that' knowledge into practice.

Taxonomies of knowing

Although many health care professionals still consider rigid investigation of empirical reality using scientific methods as the only true way of knowing, other ways of knowing have been identified. Johnson (1968) identified three types of knowledge required for practice.

- Knowledge of order
- Knowledge of disorder
- Knowledge of control

Knowledge of order: this is based on the scientific positivist approach to knowledge development, where nature is believed to be ordered and this order can be observed and described to provide us with laws and scientific theories.

Knowledge of disorder: this is represented by our awareness of events and disorders (i.e., diseases, wars, earthquakes, etc.), which threaten the well-being or survival of people and society.

Knowledge of control: here we possess knowledge that enables us to prescribe interventions that will have effects on client outcomes. This third knowledge category is very important for a practice profession like nursing.

Pierce (1957), a firm believer in the positivist way of knowing, identified seven other ways of knowing.

- knowing through being told by an authority figure
- knowing through unverified hearsay
- knowing through the experience of trial and error
- knowing indirectly through past experiences (history)
- knowing by unverified belief
- knowing through spiritual/divine understanding
- knowing through intuition.

Also a believer in the logical empirical approach, Kerlinger (1986) asserts that the way to truth is through rigorous research, involving the identification of variables within hypotheses and subjecting them to experimental manipulation. Here 'hard evidence' is required in order to be certain that something is or is not true. But Kerlinger also identified what he thought were less respectable ways of knowing.

- Knowing through tenacity
- Knowing through authority
- Knowing through a priori

Knowing through tenacity is simply knowing something because it has always been believed to be true.

Knowing though authority is knowing something because a respected or authoritative person said so.

Knowing through a priori is knowing something because reason tells you it is true (a rationalist approach).

The end result of each of these ways of knowing is knowledge; what differs is how the knowledge is acquired.

To illustrate Kerlinger's approach we could take the example of the knowledge that regular turning prevents pressure area damage to clients on bed rest. You may believe this to be true because 'it has always been done this way' (tenacity) or because the nurse lecturer told you so (authority) or because it is reasonable to assume that if a person moves themselves in bed the pressure on a particular part of the body will be lessened (a priori).

You could also have identified Kerlinger's preferred way of obtaining knowledge; you carry out regular turning procedures because you acquired the knowledge through collecting empirical data or studying the results of well-validated empirical research into pressure-relieving techniques.

Authors like Pierce and Kerlinger have the habit of building hierarchies of knowledge development. In such a scheme the scientific empiricist method is supreme and intuitive knowledge occupies a lowly position. For a practice discipline like nursing this is an inappropriate way of viewing the development of knowledge. All ways of knowing must be respected, yet all must be subject to the rigour and analysis that knowledge requires.

In 1978 Barbara Carper published an article in the first edition of the journal *Advances in Nursing Science*. The article proved to be a seminal paper on patterns of knowing in nursing. Based on earlier work she had done in 1975, Carper identified four types of knowing:

- *Empirics*: the science of nursing;
- *Aesthetics*: the art of nursing;
- *Ethics*: moral knowing;
- *Personal knowing*.

Empirics

According to Carper, 'empirics' represents knowledge that is obtained by either direct or indirect observation and measurement. In essence, it coincides with Rhyl's 'know that knowledge', Johnson's 'knowledge of order', and Kerlinger's empirical knowledge. Empirics is systematically organised into scientific principles, theories and laws for the purpose of describing, explaining and predicting phenomena of special concern to nursing. As alluded to above, much of our early research and theoretical work came under this essentially positivistic umbrella, where objectivity and generalisability were important, what Parse (1987) refers to as the 'totality paradigm'. It represents knowledge that is publicly verifiable, objective, factual and research-based. The quantifiability of empirical data allows objective measurement that yields evidence that can be replicated by multiple observers (Carper, 1992). Referring to the principle of empirics, Fogel-Keck (1994: 17) asserts that 'knowledge is based on factual information'.

Aesthetics

Empirics is a rather narrow perspective. Nursing practice may also be perceived as an art, and Carper acknowledges this in the pattern of knowing called 'aesthetics'. Such knowing finds expression in the 'art-act' (Carper, 1992). It reflects the 'know how knowledge' discussed above. Aesthetic knowledge is subjective, individual and unique. It enables us to go beyond that which is explained by existing laws and theories and accept that there are phenomena that cannot be quantified. Intuition, interpretation, understanding and valuing make up the central components of aesthetics. Here you can see the influence of historicism.

Ethics

Carper's third pattern of knowing is called 'ethics'. This is the moral component of knowing and is concerned with moral duty. This type of knowing is expressed through moral codes and ethical decision making. Practitioners set goals and undertake interventions so that clients may meet these goals. In such situations nurses often have to make choices between competing interventions. These choices and judgements may have an ethical dimension and to select the most appropriate position or action requires careful deliberation. According to Carper (1992), ethical knowledge involves the examination and evaluation of what is right and wrong and what are good, valuable and desirable end goals.

Personal knowing

If, as various theorists argue, caring is an interpersonal process (Peplau, 1952), where interaction and transaction are central (King, 1968), then we must know our own strengths and weaknesses in order to be expert practitioners. Like aesthetics, this 'personal knowing' is subjective yet is about us being aware of ourselves and how we relate to others. Most nurses are not able to prescribe medication nor do they possess an arsenal of surgical instruments: what we have is ourselves and we can use this therapeutically to make a difference to the welfare of clients. At our best, we do not perceive clients as objects but instead have a genuine relationship with those requiring help. We learn as much from a caring relationship as they do, and a good caring relationship will depend on our own self-regard. Personal knowing incorporates these issues and promotes integrity and wholeness in the client–practitioner encounter. It requires self-consciousness and active empathic participation on the part of the knower (Carper, 1992). Once again, the influence of historicism is evident in personal knowing.

Carper's work has undergone careful analysis by many authors. Kikuchi (1992), for example, agrees that every discipline should be responsible for the development of its own knowledge base, but she does not think that it can be responsible for developing the private knowledge incorporated within personal knowing and intuition. She bases her challenge on distinguishing between private knowledge and the public knowledge that can be verified and communicated.

Experienced nurses use these four patterns of knowing interchangeably. For instance, mental health nurses may use a behavioural therapy approach to care. They will be aware of the research and theoretical basis for undertaking the therapy (empirics) and they will be skilled in the practices of using positive reinforcement to encourage a change in behaviour (aesthetics). However, the issue of withholding positive reinforcers and applying sanctions with clients to alter their behaviour is a moral decision (ethics). Finally, knowing themselves and their inner resources is important in the construction of an interpersonal therapeutic relationship with the client (personal knowing).

As you reflect on these four patterns of knowing you will note the complexity of nursing knowledge. The patterns are not mutually exclusive; there is overlap, interrelation and interdependence. Such unity may be perceived as necessary for achieving mastery in what we do, where no one pattern alone should be considered sufficient (Carper, 1978).

By recognising that there are legitimate ways of knowing other than empirical knowing, Carper has made a valuable contribution to the examination of knowledge development. Chinn and Kramer (1995: 15) state that empirics, removed from the context of the whole of knowing, produces control and manipulation; ethics, removed from the context of the whole of knowing, produces rigid doctrine and insensitivity to the rights of others; aesthetics, removed from the context of the whole of knowing, produces prejudices, bigotry and lack of appreciation of meaning; and personal knowing, removed from the context of the whole of knowing, produces isolation and self-distortion.

Chinn and Kramer (1995) maintained that some form of expression is required for each of Carper's four patterns so that what is generated can be communicated. They identified 'creative' and 'expressive' dimensions. The creative dimensions are human activities that draw on the experience gained from each pattern of knowing; the expressive dimensions involve actions, words and symbols that enable what is known to be communicated. This is illustrated in Table 2.2.

Table 2.2 The creative and expressive dimensions of Carper's ways of knowing

Dimensions	Empirics	Aesthetics	Ethics	Personal
Creative	Describing	Engaging	Valuing	Opening
	Explaining	Intuiting	Clarifying	Centring
	Predicting	Envisioning	Advocating	Realising
Expressive	Facts, models	Art-act	Ethical theory	Authentic
	Theories and		Principles	genuine
	descriptions		and guidelines	self

The link between knowing and theory

But what does all this have to do with theory? Walker (1973) argues that knowledge, as fact, is gained through research, but understanding is gained by theory. Therefore, theory is an important means of achieving a rolling knowledge base in any discipline.

From Chapter 1 you will note that theory is a much abused word. Its overuse in speech has given it the status almost of cliché. People say: 'I have a theory as to why X is occurring', or 'in theory this should work', or 'theoretically, X is better than Y', or 'the theory is you place Z here' or, a more familiar statement to nurses, 'the theory–practice gap is ruining the profession'. As a word, 'theory' is common currency in ordinary conversation, but it means different things to different people.

When examining the above uses of the word 'theory' you may detect a commonality of meaning. In each case theory is synonymous with knowing or understanding. Therefore, as Folta (1971) asserts, we all theorise but we are not all theorists.

One of the main methods of communicating empirical knowing to others is through the development and testing of theory. In fact, one of the most enduring definitions of theory in nursing is 'a logically interconnected set of propositions used to describe, explain and predict a part of the empirical world' (Riehl and Roy, 1980) – an obvious reference to empiricism.

This reliance on empirical knowing as a basis for theory was probably due to the desire of some theorists to make our discipline scientific in the natural science sense, and to emulate the mostly positivistic stance taken by medicine. However, what often resulted was a greater division between clinical practice, theory and research. Considering this, Kikuchi and Simmons (1992: 2) conclude that the 'upshot was that the knowledge being developed was fragmented and ununified'.

This concentration on empirics as the desired approach to theory development and testing did not deter some theorists from using other patterns of knowing in the development of nursing theory. It is a given that theory is inescapably linked to the values and beliefs which the theorist possesses concerning the nature of human beings, nursing, the environment and health. Reed (1989) was convinced that, in order to contribute to scientific progress, theorists must incorporate a moral dimension within their theoretical reasoning where they reflect on what is good and valuable for those individuals requiring care (ethics). Similarly, how theorists generate theory and how practitioners apply theory may be influenced by their own self-awareness (personal knowing) and the skills used in practice (aesthetics).

But theory does not develop from empirics alone. Meleis (1991) maintains that theories evolve from ideas, and ideas evolve from hunches, personal experiences, insights, inspirations, intuition and the work and experience of others. The influence of ethics, aesthetics and personal knowing can be detected in the work of those theorists who focus on caring (Roach, 1992; Watson, 1985, Leininger, 1981; Boykin and Schoenhofer, 1993) and the existential theorists (Parse, 1981; Rogers, 1980; Patterson and Zderad, 1976). Rogers (1980) drew part of her theoretical influence from Polanyi's (1958) work on tacit knowledge, and by including concepts such as 'inner self' and 'essence'. Watson's theory of caring (1985) uses much of what can best be called 'personal knowledge'. Because explaining these theories in detail is beyond the remit of this book, I would refer you to the work of McQuiston and Webb (1995).

In a seminal paper, two philosophers, Dickoff and James (1968), identified four levels of theory for nursing. These will be discussed in later chapters. They are:

- Factor-isolating theory: describes and names concepts;
- Factor-relating theory: relates concepts to one another;
- Situation-relating theory: predicts interrelationship among concepts or propositions;
- Situation-producing theory: prescribes actions to reach certain outcomes.

They argued that each level of theory builds on previous levels, so that factor-isolating theory is a precursor of factor-relating theory, and so on. They also maintain that a practice discipline like nursing requires situation-producing theory, so that we could, with a degree of certainty, prescribe interventions that lead to desired results for clients. But since such prescriptive theories are based upon value premisses concerning what is the right outcome to strive for and what is the right thing to do, then ethical knowing is a central prerequisite for their development (Kim, 1989). Further, the call by Hardy (1978), for practitioners to be aware of 'the vital part that experience plays in theorising', adds support to the use of all patterns of knowing as the basis for theory.

These different ways of knowing have implications for theory testing and theory analysis. Chinn and Kramer (1995) argue that, because of the influence of aesthetics, ethics and personal knowing on nurse theorising, the resultant theories should not be analysed or critiqued using methods favoured by empiricists. To do this would denigrate these theories to a lowly position compared to biological or chemical theories on what Kerlinger (1986) would perceive as the empirical hierarchy. Robinson (1992) accepts that practitioners will continue to apply natural science knowledge in some aspects of their practice, but she states that care is a social process and has to be analysed using tools different from those found in natural sciences.

Nursing science

In the 1950s, Peplau was the first nurse to use the term 'nursing science' (Peplau, 1987). Fogel-Keck (1994: 17) defines nursing science as 'that body of knowledge germane to the discipline of nursing, plus the processes and methodologies used to gain that knowledge'. Echoing this, Powers and Knapp (1995: 140) define science as an activity that combines research (the advancement of knowledge) with theory (explanation of knowledge). Therefore, in most definitions of science, the body of knowledge referred to is empirical knowledge. In Chapter 1 research was perceived as the tool of science and theories as the products of science. Both of these will now be examined in turn.

Research as a basis for knowledge development

In 1968, Johnson made a clarion call for nurses to identify the phenomena which had relevance for nursing as a distinct discipline and to ask questions in a way that would be different from those asked by other disciplines. It was only by doing this, she believed, that nursing would acquire the body of knowledge needed for its practice. Earlier, Rogers (1961: 43) stated that 'theoretical knowledge is dependent on research'. Therefore, in order to discover new knowledge and verify existing knowledge, various methods of enquiry must be employed.

Research is defined as 'rigorous and systematic enquiry conducted on a scale and using methods commensurate with the issue to be investigated, and designed to lead to more generalised contributions to knowledge' (Department of Health, 1994: 37).

Generalisation is invariably associated with randomised controlled trials and most researchers who use a qualitative approach would not claim that their data are generalisable. Therefore, like most definitions of research it is possible, in Department of Health terminology, to see plainly the influence of empiricism. As referred to above, the need to confirm and verify takes precedence within this approach. The result is hard numerical data representing reality that are then often accepted as truth and enter the knowledge base of the profession.

Nurses, in attempting to gain academic respect with other longer established professions, adopted the positivist approach over other forms of enquiry when developing and testing theories. Those nurses who did pioneer other methods of enquiry, relating to understanding rather than control, were seldom given the recognition accorded to the former. But to think that research can only be empiric and scientific (in the natural science usage of the term) is incorrect. It is noteworthy that while nurses were adopting the positivistic approach to research, philosophers such as Kuhn (1970), Suppe (1977) and Laudan (1977) were realising the shortcomings of these methods and had already moved on to supporting other ways of developing knowledge.

The following illustrates the importance that one leading nurse placed on the empiricist approach to nursing enquiry:

1   Specify, define and classify the concepts used in describing the phenomena of the field;
2   Develop statements or propositions that propose how two or more concepts are related;
3   Specify how all the propositions are related to each other in a systematic way.

(Jacox 1974)

According to Gortner (1993: 479), Jacox subsequently acknowledged that her early writings were 'unduly influenced by positivism'. It seemed as if nurses were always at least one step behind in their search for and use of methods of enquiry. According to Emden (1991), this may still be the case: while contemporary nurse researchers are extolling the virtues of hermeneutics as an approach to knowledge development, philosophers are no longer granting it the attention they once did.

Acceptance of new patterns of knowledge development in nursing has gradually led to the realisation that new methods are required to build and test this new knowledge. Miller (1989) states that, since nursing involves caring and nurturing within a social context, any attempt to investigate or teach it using methods developed in the natural sciences is inappropriate. It has become clear that such methods can neither ask nor answer many of the questions that are germane to nursing practice. In the mid-1970s the traditional positivistic approach was found wanting: as a result, many nurse researchers deserted it and, following in the footsteps of social scientists, they embraced other approaches. Nurse theorists too began to reject the empirical pattern of knowing and sought, from the work of philosophers, new scientific approaches by which to develop and test their work. Examples of this quest for research approaches to suit their theory include Parse (1981), who favoured a phenomenological approach, Benner (1983), hermeneutics, and Watson (1985), qualitative methodologies. (Parse (1987) is a good source of further information on these approaches.)

None the less, the contribution of the positivistic research approach to nursing knowledge cannot be denied, and it should not be rejected completely. In Britain there have been some very good research projects which, although having their basis in the experimental positivist tradition, have contributed substantially to nursing knowledge (Tierney, 1973; Boore, 1978; Metcalf, 1982; Pearson, 1985; Armitage, 1990; McKenna, 1992).

A useful way to view research methods is to see them as a bag of tools. When you come across a clinical problem, you reach into the bag and extract a method. If the method is inappropriate for the problem identified then another method is selected. It may be just as inappropriate to select a qualitative method from the historicism stable as a quantitative method from the rationalist or empiricist stable: it depends on the topic or problem to be investigated. But, regardless of which method is used to generate knowledge, as alluded to above, the key research skills have to do with being rigorous and systematic.

New methods of research do not just happen: they are the products of much philosophic thought and discussion. The initiators of new methods ask what it is like to be human, are our species merely objects which can be studied in a detached manner by detached investigators or are they holistic individuals whose totality is greater than the sum of their parts? The answers to these questions lead nursing scholars to seek new ways of studying human beings. One broad approach was based on what Wilhelm Dilthey (1833–1911) referred to as 'human science' . The reader will note that it emanates from the historicist philosophy of science.

Human science values subjective opinion, beliefs, personal

knowledge, descriptions of experiences and feelings, many of which are not amenable to objective verification. Human science also recognises the effect the researcher and the research participants/respondents have on what is being researched. Intuition, understanding, reflection, meanings and experiences are central components of the human science approach. Within human science the participants' 'lived experiences' are the core of explanations and meanings about things, and are interpreted by the participants not by outsiders. Humans are perceived as whole people and breaking them down into components is seen as dehumanising. Conversations and interactions require interpretation, and uncovering patterns in these is an appropriate goal of human science. Meleis (1995) refers to research in human science as the *perceived view* as opposed to the *received view* of empiricism (see Table 2.3).

Table 2.3 The received view versus the perceived view (after Meleis, 1995)

Received view	Perceived view
Objective	Subjective
Deduction	Induction
One truth	Multiple truths
Validation and replication	Trends and patterns
Justification	Discovery
Test theories	Evaluate theories
Prediction and control	Description and understanding
Particulars	Patterns
Reductionism	Holism
Generalisation	Individualism
Empirical positivism	Historicism

Chinn and Kramer (1995) accept the importance of both views for the development of knowledge for practice. In traditional science an attempt is made to study the whole through looking at its parts, while in human science an attempt is made to study the whole as it appears. In traditional science, knowledge is developed to describe, to explain and to predict; in human science, knowledge is developed to understand. In traditional science, theory is developed through defining, analysing and synthesising concepts and propositions; in human science, theory is developed through description and interpretation. Traditional science is directed towards uncovering cause-and-effect relationships and generalisations; human science is directed towards creating knowledge from common meanings, patterns and themes in descriptions. Both seek empirical honesty through methodological rigour (Smith, 1994: 51).

In 1987 Rosemary Parse argued that there were two central paradigms within nursing. More recently, William Cody (1995) supports this notion. The two paradigms are the *totality paradigm* (loosely equivalent to the received view of science) and the *simultaneity paradigm* (loosely equivalent to the perceived view of science). More will be written about these two paradigms in later chapters.

It is heartening that nurses are beginning to accept and use methods of enquiry other than the empiricist approach. This development should have a powerful effect on identifying a body of knowledge that has particular relevance to patient care. In this way 'know that' and 'know why' knowledge can enrich the 'know how' knowledge and vice versa.

It is important to note dissenting voices. Susan Gadow (1990) does not think human science goes far enough in explaining how best to develop nursing knowledge. She believes the researcher should leave the personal alone and leave experience alone because there is no way to summarise (reduce) a life, a culture or any human situation. Qualitative research is no better than quantitative here, in that it treats experience as data. She appears to argue that quantitative researchers may be more honest because they are 'up front' in calling the subject the object of their study (cited in Smith, 1994).

Developing nursing knowledge through reasoning

Inductive reasoning

Every day practitioners deal with client phenomena (see Chapter 1). By taking note of patterns and commonality in those phenomena that are of special interest to nursing, it is possible to build up a body of knowledge. This is referred to as 'inductive reasoning'. The early empiricists favoured this method when developing theory. However, qualitative research approaches from the historicist school of philosophy also use induction to generate theory ('know that' knowledge) from practice ('know how' knowledge).

Deductive reasoning

In contrast to inductive reasoning, deductive reasoning involves moving from the general to the specific. You will note above that René Descartes favoured it as a key component of rationalism. From Chapter 1 you will remember that traditionally deductive reasoning involves the use of three propositions (two premises and one conclusion). In physics, premises are also called 'axioms' or 'postulates' and conclusions are also called 'theorems'. In deductive reasoning a conclusion follows from one or more statements that are taken as true. Aristotle (384–322 BC) perfected this form of deductive argument, calling it a 'syllogism'. The most famous example is shown in Box 2.3:

Box 2.3 **Aristotelian syllogism**		
All men are mortal	(1st premise)	(axiom 1 or postulate 1)
Socrates is a man	(2nd premise) OR	(axiom 2 or postulate 2)
Therefore Socrates is mortal	(conclusion)	(theorem)

You can see that if the premises remained the same but I changed the conclusion to read 'Socrates is not mortal', then the deductive reasoning would be faulty. Similarly, if one of the premises was reversed, the unchanged conclusion would be wrong and the reasoning would once again be faulty. The importance of identifying faulty reasoning is specified when analysing the internal structure of theories in Chapter 7.

You could reverse the example and make it inductive reasoning. Here a series of discrete observations about a phenomenon is followed by a conclusion, as in Box 2.4:

Box 2.4 Example of inductive reasoning

Confucius is a man and is mortal	(1st premise)
Socrates is a man and is mortal	(2nd premise)
Hannibal is a man and is mortal	(3rd premise)
Therefore all men are mortal	(conclusion)

Deductive reasoning in nursing normally starts with an established theory and this (or part of it) is tested in the real world of practice to see if it can be disproved – remember the paper boat.

Retroductive reasoning

Whether theories should be developed deductively or inductively is seen as a false argument by Jacox and Webster (1992). They state that some theorists will use a more deductive or a more inductive approach than others, but all theory construction includes both. It is not an either/or issue.

Many authors agree that induction and deduction are often used together in a research study. This is referred to as 'retroduction'. An example of this type of research would be that of Boore (1978). Boore used an experimental design to test the theory that providing information to pre-operative patients would reduce their stress levels post-operatively. Since a specific theory was being tested and applied, the method used was deduction. However, the results of this study led to new practices in how patients are prepared for surgery and a 'practice theory' of pre-operative preparation was developed. Here, Boore was using induction where experiences within the research setting led to the development of a new, more clinically specific, theory.

Summary

Nursing knowledge and the research to generate and test that knowledge have been linked with positivism. However, there is a wealth of literature to suggest that nurses use other ways of knowing and that these do not fit neatly within the empirical framework. Many of these patterns of knowing are being incorporated within contemporary theorising. This has led to new theoretical perspectives. There has also been the realisation that new research methods must be formulated to test and develop theory of this nature. The positivist approach may still have a place, but its importance has diminished greatly in recent years.

While empiricism continues to play a major role in the development of knowledge and theory, historicism – with its emphasis on theory generation – is being seen as a worthwhile endeavour. Both approaches are necessary. Similarly, it is also possible for a researcher to obtain a richer perspective on certain phenomena by using both inductive and deductive approaches in the same study in the form of retroduction.

Chapter 3
Building theory through concept analysis

In Chapter 1 the relationship between the terms 'phenomenon', 'concept', 'proposition' and 'theory' was discussed. Chapter 2 dealt with how different philosophies of science can be used to extend nursing's knowledge base. In essence, theory is composed of conceptual bricks joined together in various systematic ways by statements called propositions. Because of this, to understand theory one must first understand concepts. To try to build or use a theory without having a clear understanding of the conceptual 'building blocks' would be to lay faulty theoretical foundations for the discipline of nursing.

Concepts, whether incorporated within a theory or not, explain and describe phenomena. Therefore, if the concept is unclear, its role in the propositional statements that seek to explain, describe or predict is questionable. This chapter aims to demonstrate how readers can clarify and analyse concepts in order to achieve understanding. Many of the concepts used in nursing, such as caring, empathy, self-esteem, frailty, etc., are abstract and nebulous and, as Janice Morse (1995: 32) states, 'there is a vast amount of conceptual exploration yet to be accomplished'. She continues, 'Because the theoretical base is the foundation of nursing research and practice, at this time the most urgent need for methodologic development in nursing exists in the area of conceptual inquiry.'

At the outset it has to be stated that there is the potential for confusion: concepts make up theory, yet concepts used by nurses often come from existing theory. Kaplan (1964) referred to this as the 'paradox of conceptualisation'. He realised that good concepts are essential to formulate good theory, but you also need good theory to provide you with good concepts. Therefore, the better our concepts, the better the theory we can generate with them and in turn the better the concepts available for future theory development.

Earlier, we defined concepts as representations of phenomena that we perceive and experience in our environment. However, when nurses and non-nurses observe the same phenomena they may perceive and experience them differently. Concepts used in a professional way by members of a discipline are normally called 'second order concepts' (Moody, 1990). This means that the same words are used differently within the profession than they would be by non-professionals. What a member of the public would understand by the terms 'dimension' or 'becoming' would be different from that of a Rogerian (Rogers, 1980) or Parsean (Parse, 1981) scholar. Within nursing too, perceptions may differ concerning the same clinical phenomena; concept analysis should reduce this conceptual confusion.

From Chapter 1, you may recall that concepts vary along a continuum from concrete (sometimes called empirical or descriptive concepts) to abstract (sometimes called constructs). Another illustration of this would be the following: as they grow older, children know that an animal that barks, has hair, a tail and four legs is, more than likely, a dog. This is a very concrete concept. However, the child may call the dog Lassie, the child's parents may call it a household pet, the neighbours may call it a mongrel, another member of the family may refer to the dog as a loyal companion or man's best friend and the veterinary surgeon may refer to it as a member of the canine species. Although these terms are referring to the same animal, they represent concepts at different points on the concrete–abstract continuum.

Moody (1990) identified three levels of concepts:

- Global concepts
- Middle-range concepts
- Empirical concepts

Global concepts: these are those represented by the metaparadigm: person, nursing environment and health.

Middle-range concepts: these involve such concepts as self-care, energy fields, adaptation, etc., and may be related to one or more of the global concepts.

Empirical concepts: these are more precise and include measurable concepts such as hours of sleep, body temperature, etc. These may be subsumed under the middle-range concepts of adaptation or self-care.

According to Moody (1990), in order to extend the knowledge base of nursing, a concept analysis needs to focus on concepts relevant to the metaparadigm. The reasons for this are clear: there are many concepts of specific relevance to nursing which are used inconsistently and lead to confusion among patients and staff. Nursing may be better served if the meaning of such concepts was clarified rather than time being spent analysing concepts which have more in common with the metaparadigms of other disciplines. In the latter case, the nurse would only be extending the knowledge base of the other discipline.

Notwithstanding this, it is possible that the outcome of an analysis undertaken by a nurse would be different from the outcome of an analysis carried out by a member of another professional discipline. Therefore, concepts borrowed from other disciplines may be reconstituted through analysis in order to generate meanings appropriate for nursing.

Why undertake concept analysis?

Concept analysis enables us to refine and define a concept that has originated in practice, research or theory. It helps us to differentiate it from similar and dissimilar concepts. The end result is a way of reliably checking or operationalising the existence of that concept in nursing practice. Therefore, concept analysis is a core activity in the development of theory. In fact, according to Dickoff and James (1968), the first level of theorising is 'factor-isolating theory', which is the naming and clarification of concepts. This seems to indicate that the end result of concept analysis is descriptive theory.

Many authors have identified methods of analysing concepts (Wilson, 1969; Smith and Medin, 1981; Norris, 1970; Moody, 1990; Rodgers, 1994, Walker and Avant, 1995; Morse, 1995). Chinn and

Kramer (1995) describe the process as a technique or mental activity that requires critical approaches to uncovering subtle elements of meaning that can be embedded in concepts. The process is a highly deliberate and disciplined activity.

The various authors referred to above identify a variety of steps that you may follow in order to analyse a concept. I propose to use a mixture of Walker and Avant (1995) and Chinn and Kramer (1995), both of whose works use Wilson's (1969) criteria as an organisational template. I also plan to take cognisance of Rodgers (1994) and Morse (1995), who both berate Wilson's method and suggest a more qualitative approach to concept analysis.

Step 1: select the concept of interest

As with most new processes, the first step may be the most difficult. A concept may be selected which originates from an intuitive feeling or an area of concern. The best concept analyses tend to have their roots in clinical phenomena. This helps to bridge the theory–practice gap in that the end result has more credibility and relevance for practice. The concept can also lead to the development of theory which can be more easily used and tested in practice.

Meleis (1991) suggests that while giving care a practitioner's attention may be attracted to a particular phenomenon. She refers to this as 'attention grabbing' and states that it can occur concurrently during the care episode or retrospectively when the nurse is reflecting about the care given. The attention-grabbing phase is followed by the 'attention-giving' phase. This is a more active and deliberate process.

Answers to the following attention-giving questions may help to clarify the hunch that the nurse has about the phenomenon of interest. For example, the nurse may ask: 'why do patients get angry with their spouse during visiting time?', or 'what is it that happens when patients decide not to attend a clinic?', or 'what are the properties of pre-operative anxiety?'. Observing a bereaved relative coming to get support from a staff member who had looked after the deceased patient is a beginning observation that may evolve into a phenomenon. As similar observations occur the observer can ask questions, read and reflect.

Meleis (1991) would appear to agree with Moody's assertion that nursing phenomena should form the focus of the analysis. To ensure that the nursing focus is not inadvertently ignored, Meleis urges the nurse to persist with probing questions:

- How is the phenomenon related to nursing's body of knowledge?
- Would understanding the phenomenon contribute to better understanding of a patient care issue?
- How would questions relating to the phenomenon be significant for nursing?

Once these questions have been answered, the nurse labels the phenomenon with a word or a short phrase. Labels should be precise, used consistently when referring to the phenomenon, contain one cardinal idea and be fundamental to the definition/description of the phenomenon (Meleis, 1991). As stated in Chapter 1, this label is a concept.

In your everyday clinical work, you may notice that ward sisters are able to predict client mishaps before they occur and without knowing precisely how they are able to do this. The concept 'intuition' is the term you would select to describe this phenomenon. From other clinical experiences you may also be interested in clarifying what the concepts 'loss', 'loneliness', 'compassion' or 'spirituality' really mean.

Moody (1990) suggests that it may be helpful to categorise the concept requiring analysis within the metaparadigm. For instance, the concept 'well-being' may be subsumed under health; 'identity' or 'body image' under person; 'caring' or 'empathy' under nursing; and 'energy field' under environment.

Perhaps the best rule of thumb is to select a concept that represents phenomena that interest or intrigue you. For the first analysis you undertake it may also be a good idea to avoid broad concepts: for instance, if you were to select 'communications' as a concept you would find it extremely difficult to identify manageable indicators which are representative of this concept. Paradoxically, it is suggested that the concept to be analysed should be abstract enough to retain its meaning when it is removed from highly specific situations, while it should also be precise enough that its boundaries are identifiable (Walker and Avant, 1995; Moody, 1990).

The additional reading list at the end of this chapter will show that a range of concepts can be selected for analyses. These include: sorrow, hope, intuition, caring, grief, restlessness, trust, quality of life, dignity, comfort, feeling, burnout, etc.

Step 2: define the aims of the analysis

There are many reasons why you would wish to undertake a concept analysis. You may want to reduce a complex concept to its component parts for examination of its internal structure and, by so doing, increase its explanatory power. Concept analysis also offers the opportunity to examine and clarify confusing or unclear concepts in an existing theory and provide the basis for operational definitions, for refining and generating research questions and hypotheses and as a foundation stone for critical thinking. It can also allow the operationalisation of variables for testing a theory or hypothesis through a research study.

Not only does concept analysis refine the meaning of ambiguous concepts, it also clarifies overused concepts, differentiates a concept from other similar yet different concepts and lays the foundation for theory development. The outcome of a successful concept analysis is the identification of empirical indicators to reliably inform us of the presence or absence of the concept.

Step 2 should provide a good rationale as to why you are undertaking the process at all. You may be able to provide a research-based justification for selecting a particular concept. Government reports and health care strategies may highlight old concepts being used in new ways (quality of care) or new concepts being used to denote old ideas (nursing diagnoses). It is recommended that a short rationale is constructed to justify why a particular concept should be analysed.

In most cases, the prime purpose for undertaking an analysis is to elucidate and to create conceptual meaning for a clinical phenomenon. For instance, the term 'caring' is often used in many confusing ways, and an analysis of this concept would tell you what it is and what it is not. You may also wish to take a central concept from a theory and seek to understand it better (e.g., adaptation, becoming, self-care).

Step 2 will set the parameters for later steps in the process. For instance, if your purpose was to investigate fear or hopelessness among coronary care patients then this will guide you towards those indicators and attributes identified as an aid to recognising and investigating these concepts.

Step 3: identify meanings of the concept

This step involves trawling the literature to find as many pertinent meanings of the concept as possible. Depending on the concept, this could be a major undertaking and, as a result, the search should be limited to the purpose identified in Step 2. The search will provide you with a range of different ways in which the concept is thought about and used. Walker and Avant (1995) suggest that you should cast your net as wide as possible in seeking meanings for the concept. Rodgers (1994) also recommends sampling a range of uses, stating that this increases the rigour of the analysis.

If the concept was 'caring', you will note that it could be perceived as a noun or an adjective, whereas 'care' could be a verb. 'Care' could also mean caution or attention or protection. It is a good idea to keep searching until you reach the stage of 'diminishing returns', where no new meanings are being uncovered.

Dictionaries will give you information on the Latin or Greek origins of the concept of interest. Thesauri will provide you with a range of similar concepts. However, definitions are often unclear and ambiguous, so simply providing a list of definitions of a concept should not be construed as undertaking an analysis.

It is also recommended that you examine what theorists or researchers have said about the concept. You do not have to confine your search to nursing, but may include all those who have attempted to use the concept within their theory or study.

There are other sources that may give you an insight into the use of the concept. These include professional, popular, classical and philosophical literature, poetry, books of quotations, music, paintings, cartoons and photographs. The film *Philadelphia* may be an excellent source of information on the concept 'loss', *Schindler's*

List may provide a unique view of the concept 'sorrow'; and *The Silence of the Lambs* may give a different perspective on the concept 'fear'. You could also ask colleagues and family what they understand by the concept. Whether or not you use all these sources will depend on the concept and the purpose of the analysis. For concepts of interest to nursing, such as caring, empathy, dignity, identity, etc., the above sources may well provide valuable insights.

For Step 3 it must be remembered that the objective is to uncover meaning, not to describe, explain or predict relationships between the concept of interest and other similar or dissimilar concepts. This is a more advanced form of theorising and may indeed be undertaken at a later stage as a result of concept analysis (see below).

Step 4: determine the defining attributes

The meanings of the concept identified in Step 3 explicate the particular characteristics of the concept that occur again and again. These represent its hallmarks, what Walker and Avant (1995) refer to as the 'defining attributes' of the concept. In essence, the defining attributes distinguish the concept (as envisaged in Step 2) from similar or related concepts. By isolating the defining attributes, the 'semantic space' that the concept shares with similar concepts is reduced (Moody, 1990).

For each concept there may be a list of several defining attributes, but extra superfluous defining attributes should not be added just because the list appears too short. It is better to have three or four defining attributes that really characterise the concept well, than to have many that are only tangentially related to the concept. A defining attribute of caring may be 'providing for another', a defining attribute for empathy may be 'demonstrating concern', and a defining attribute of attachment may be 'visual contact'.

Kim (1983) argues that when nurses are undertaking conceptual analysis they should ensure that the defining attributes are examined for their degree of consistency with nursing's perspective. She argues that such an approach will help focus the analysis on the phenomena of specific concern to the discipline.

The defining attributes play a key role in differentiating the concept being analysed from dissimilar concepts. One strategy to see if this is the case is to take each defining attribute in turn and challenge a colleague to identify a contrary example of the concept that does not include that particular defining attribute. If the defining attribute also applies to the contrary example, then it is an imprecise attribute for the concept being analysed and it can be dropped from the list. Moody (1990) calls this the 'test for necessity', where failure to pass means that more work has to be done to identify the defining attributes.

The 'test of sufficiency' should also be applied. Here, the entire list of defining attributes is considered and, if a contrary case can be identified that meets all the attributes, then an essential attribute has been omitted.

Moody (1990) gives the example of an analysis of a right-angled triangle (a concrete concept). She identified the following three defining attributes:

1   Two-dimensional geometric figure;
2   composed of three sides;
3   the sum of the internal angles equals 180 degrees.

Since Attribute 1 could be applied to any geometric figure, the 'test of necessity' indicates that it is not a necessary attribute for defining a right-angled triangle: this attribute can be removed from the list. The other two attributes pass the 'test of necessity'.

Applying the 'test of sufficiency' to the remaining two attributes it is noted that other types of triangle meet these criteria (e.g., an equilateral triangle). It is obvious that some key attributes which differentiate this concept from other similar concepts are missing. Clearly, attributes indicating that one of the angles must be 90 degrees and the other two angles must be 45 degrees each should be included as defining attributes.

While the tests of necessity and sufficiency help in the identification of defining attributes, it must be remembered that the concepts of interest to nurses are not as concrete as right-angled triangles. While the two tests may be useful in the analysis of abstract concepts, the borders between what is a defining attribute and what is not for these concepts may not be as clear-cut. Therefore, the identification of defining attributes is an inexact science, but it is valuable in that it does yield important information for the clarification of concepts for clinical and research purposes.

McCance (1996) undertook a concept analysis of caring. From a wealth of literature (Step 3 above) she identified the following defining attributes of caring:

- Serious attention
- Concern
- Providing for
- Regard, respect, or liking

Step 5: identify a model case

Definitions from dictionaries and thesauri give the analyst an insight into the concept of interest. However, it has to be admitted that for abstract concepts, such as those found in nursing, the identification of model and alternative cases is often a more valuable way of gaining insight. A model case is a pure example of the concept being used and should include all the defining attributes. It may be written in one or two paragraphs indicating a hypothetical case, an extract from the literature illustrating a real-life event or, preferably, a clinical example that accurately describes the concept. Rodgers (1994) argues that by providing a real-life example that includes all the defining attributes, a model case enhances the degree of clarification and credibility of the concept.

Considering model cases, Wilson (1969) maintains that when you view a model case you can say with absolute certainty that if this is not X (the concept) then nothing is. You have probably realised that it is easier to construct model cases with concrete concepts than with abstract concepts. A rule of thumb is that there must be no contradictions between the model case and the defining attributes. In other words, a model case must include all the defining attributes.

McCance (1996) presented the model case shown in Box 3.1 to illustrate the concept 'caring':

> **Box 3.1 Case model: 'caring'**
>
> Mr Cook was in the terminal stages of congestive heart fail-
> ure. He had two myocardial infarctions. He was alone, his
> family were out of town. We knew he wasn't doing well . . .
> When I touched his hand and introduced myself . . . he
> squeezed my hand and began to talk . . . I sat on his bed, and
> he reached out and held my hand. He talked to me about his
> life, about his family, and the things he wanted to do but was-
> n't able to . . . I ignored everything else that was going on in
> the unit at that time: and it was busy. I pulled the curtains
> around one side of the bed because there was some activity
> coming from that side. I just sat and listened as he spoke.
>
> (Ford, 1990: 160, cited in McCance, 1996)

Each of the four defining attributes identified by McCance above
were included in this model case.

Step 6: identify alternative cases

Alternative cases are identified to provide examples of what is *not*
the concept. To do this often helps clarify with certainty what *is* the
concept. Alternative cases include contrary cases, related cases,
borderline cases, invented cases and illegitimate cases.

Contrary case

This case represents what is *not* the concept being analysed, and
this would be obvious to most people. Viewing this case it is possible to say with certainty that whatever this case is, it is not an
example of the concept. Chinn and Kramer (1995) warn against
simply identifying an opposite case to the model case. They suggest
that this does not add any significant new information to the analysis. When examining the concept of 'caring', a contrary case would
be an example of an interaction where a nurse was consciously
harming a client. With some of the more nebulous concepts in

nursing, a contrary case may be easier to identify than a model case and may subsequently help in the identification of a model case.

McCance (1996) presents the contrary case shown in Box 3.2 in her analysis of 'caring'. It is a description of a nurse given by a patient with lupus erythematosis.

Box 3.2 Contrary case: 'caring'

She was always in a hurry, she didn't have time to talk or even if she had time she didn't really seem to want to talk. Her body language let me know she wasn't interested in what I had to say. All she was here to do was to perform her duty and go home. She stood at a distance, she didn't even come close. She made me feel I have some kind of illness and it might rub off on her. When I was talking to her she wouldn't look at me directly. When I would ask her a question she would be snappy – even on the defensive side. She wasn't interested in the person as a whole. She would cut me off short and she talked in such a rush. She never would say when she'd be back. I was not at ease. I was uncomfortable. I became depressed by not being able to talk. I felt I had to keep my mouth shut.

The nurse in the above case shows no concern, provides no help or comfort to the patient, is in no way present or attentive and makes no attempt to get to know this patient and what is important to them. Within McCance's analysis, the defining attributes are missing here, and this is a clear example of what caring is *not*.

Related case

In a related case all the defining attributes are missing but the concept is still seen as similar in meaning to the concept being analysed. Related cases may represent concepts that are often confused with the concept under study. For instance, 'innovation' is sometimes misconstrued with change, the concept 'stress' with burnout, 'fear' with anxiety, 'adaptation' with coping, and the concept 'comfort' is often confused with care. Using these concepts as related cases demonstrates examples that are similar to the concept of interest but differ from it when you examine them closely.

Borderline case

This example is very similar to a model case but some of the defining attributes are missing. This inclusion of some of the defining attributes in a borderline case also differentiates it from a related case. Identifying borderline cases helps to clarify the attributes which are an essential prerequisite of the model case and helps to reduce the blurring of the boundaries between cases. Meleis (1991) recommends what she calls 'analogising'. Here, the concept is compared to similar concepts which have been researched well and studied more extensively so that the examination of the better understood concept may shed more light on what the new concept is. McCance (1996) presents the example of a borderline case of 'caring' in Box 3.3 (see p. 68).

It can be seen that two of the defining attributes identified by McCance above are missing from this case. Defining attributes 'serious attention' and 'regard for' are missing in this case while 'providing for' and 'concern' are present.

Invented case

This refers to a case that takes the concept out of its normal context and places it in an invented, out-of-the-ordinary, situation. Imagination may run riot here. For instance, subterranean humanoids foraging in the pit of a volcano gathering sustaining food for their offspring may be an example of the concept 'caring'. According to Moody (1990), invented cases are particularly useful when a concept describes an unfamiliar phenomenon or when clarity is needed for a familiar concept whose existence is often overlooked under normal circumstances. The analyst may also identify an invented alternative case, in other words, an invented case that is not caring.

Box 3.3 Borderline case: 'caring'

Jim Smith was forty-five years old when I met him . . . He was admitted to the cardiopulmonary unit where I was working. The patient had an eight-hour history of slurred speech and blurred vision. The symptoms had cleared up prior to his admission and he was now admitted for a diagnostic workup . . . He was worked up for transitory ischaemic arterial spasm. Four days later he went home with a negative workup. Two days after that he was readmitted after having a seizure at home. I was on holiday at the time, and by the time I had returned he had a diagnosis of metatistic lung cancer.

I do not know how he responded to the initial diagnosis – when I returned, I didn't go in to see him for a couple of days. I was really frightened about seeing him because I did not know what to say or do. He made it easy for me, and I did begin working with him again, concentrating on teaching him about chemotherapy and radiotherapy. I felt I was teaching him a lot, but actually he taught me. One day he said to me, "You are doing an OK job Mary, but I can tell that every time you walk in that door you are walking out."

He was right. He had developed so much meaning in his illness and life that I was not relating to. This man had really expanded the context of his life into areas where I could have been effective, had I had some understanding.

(Benner and Wrubel, 1989: 16, cited in McCance, 1996)

Illegitimate case

This type of case is a real-life example of the concept being used inappropriately for the purpose of the analysis. For example, if the concept being analysed was 'attachment', an illegitimate case could be an attachment for a portable drill or saw. Similarly, if the concept was 'curing', an illegitimate case may involve a butcher curing bacon.

Step 7: identify antecedents and consequences

This step is useful in that it gives an indication of the purpose of the analysis and the clinical arena in which the concept is normally used. Antecedents are those events that precede the occurrence of the concept. Antecedent is not synonymous with causality. An antecedent may contribute to the occurrence of the concept, it may be associated with its occurrence or it may need to be present for the concept to be present. Walker and Avant (1995) maintain that something cannot be an antecedent and a defining attribute at the same time. McCance (1996) identified the following antecedents of caring: 'a respect for persons', 'an amount of time' and 'the intention to care'. You can see that 'respect for persons' could be confused as a defining attribute for caring. However, in order to be a defining attribute it would have to be respect for the person(s) being cared for rather than respect for persons in general.

Consequences are those events or outcomes that happen after the occurrence of the concept. If the concept was anxiety, an antecedent may be bad news or a request to go to the chief executive's office. Consequences of anxiety may be physiological changes and avoidance behaviour. Once more, care must be taken that the consequences are not seen as defining attributes for the concept. Well-being, both physical and mental, was seen as one of the consequences of caring as analysed by McCance (1996).

Step 8: consider context and values

Morse (1995) criticises Walker and Avant (1995) for not taking account of context in their concept analysis scheme. This is a valid criticism and the importance of contextual issues in concept development will be dealt with here. It has been alluded to above that concepts have different meanings depending on the context in which they are used. For example, caring in an intensive care unit may be perceived differently from caring in an elderly rehabilitation unit or in Africa compared to Japan.

Contextually, language and culture play a major role in how concepts are viewed. The concept 'snow' is an example: the Eskimo has numerous words to denote snow, whereas an African may only have one. In Irish Gaelic there are several different words that mean 'love', but each is slightly different and gives a unique perspective on the concept. As a result, Gaelic songs and poems about love lose meaning when translated into English. Even within English-speaking countries, you may note that different regions have different dialects or use colloquialisms that give a variety of meanings to the concept of interest. For instance, to one group of people the concept 'bread' may mean a loaf, to another group it may refer to money and to yet another group it may designate a desired possession as in 'the bread of life'.

Values and beliefs are also important considerations. Dependency may be seen as a normal social need in some communities but as a burden on society in others. Clients' self-care may be seen as important and valuable by some nurses but as upsetting to the ward routine by others.

Step 9: identify empirical indicators

These are explicit referents for measuring or appraising the existence of the concept. This step is often referred to as the operationalisation of a concept. In other words, armed with these indicators, it would be possible to see 'beyond a shadow of a doubt' if the concept was present. In some cases, the empirical indicators will be the same as the defining attributes identified in Step 4 above. However, according to Walker and Avant (1995) sometimes the concept is so abstract that the defining attributes are also abstract, and therefore would not make good empirical indicators. For instance, a defining attribute for care could be 'providing for', while an empirical indicator for care may be actually physically interacting with someone. Such indicators are useful in research and practice because they can provide criteria by which a concept can be measured.

Empirical indicators are relatively easy to identify for concrete concepts. However, it is possible to identify such indicators even for abstract concepts. Chinn and Kramer (1995), for instance, analysed 'mothering'. They identified several empirical indicators, two of which are:

● The person who receives mothering must be physically touched by the mothering person;

● Some positive feeling must be experienced by the mothering person and by the person who receives the mothering.

The foregoing stepwise concept analysis has not been without its detractors. The identification of empirical indicators and the perception of linearity in the nine steps give the impression of quantification and reductionism and this has led to it being criticised by Rodgers (1994) and Morse (1995) as being positivistic and constraining. These authors argue that the concepts of interest to nursing should be analysed using a more qualitative approach. However, it must be stated that, although concept analysis is presented here as a linear series of steps, this is often not the case in reality. It may become an iterative process and, particularly when a person becomes skilled in this process, several of the steps may be dealt with simultaneously. Also, the cases cited refer to real-life situations extracted from the literature. Furthermore, Step 8 has been introduced to account for the influence of culture and context.

Another criticism levelled at concept analysis is that individuals know all along what the term means and that the exercise is futile. Morse (1995: 32) argues that the stepwise approach 'simplifies the complexity of concept development and often produces trivial and insignificant results'. This may be an erroneous assumption since the accusation depends on the concept selected for analysis and how the steps are used. As alluded to above, the many abstract concepts encountered in nursing can lead to misunderstanding and confusion. At its best, concept analysis is an intellectual exercise that requires creative and critical thinking and leads to clarification and understanding of the building blocks of knowledge.

Considering Morse's (1995) criticism of the traditional approach to concept analysis, her qualitative alternative is presented here. She admits surprise that methods of concept analysis have only recently moved from reliance on published work as examples of model and alternative cases to the use of actual real-life situations presented in the form of qualitative data. She calls for the use of actual data or the use of secondary analysis of data in the literature rather than 'invented cases' and brief accounts that lack detail.

Morse states that concept analysis should commence with a comprehensive review of the literature. The review should include dictionaries, clinical articles, research articles and autobiographic experiential accounts. Depending on what is found in the literature, Morse recommends six different strategies.

1 If the concept remains unclear after the literature review, undertake concept development

Concept development is composed of three phases:

- identifying the attributes of the concept;
- verifying the attributes;
- identifying manifestations of the concept.

Identifying the attributes of the concept

According to Morse (1995), this phase involves the identification of an incident or event which is considered to be an exemplar of the concept. This differs from the 'model case' approach of Walker and Avant (1995) in that the exemplar has to be a real-life event or incident. Morse even suggests that the analyst should exclude previous knowledge and assumptions, as would be the case in a qualitative phenomenological study. All concepts have particular attributes or characteristics and by closely examining the exemplar it should be possible to extract the concept's key attributes. From an exemplar concerning a family caught in a snowdrift, Morse identified the following attributes for the concept 'hope':

- A realistic initial assessment of the predicament or threat;
- The envisioning of alternatives and the setting of goals;
- A bracing for negative outcomes;
- A realistic assessment of personal resources and of external conditions and resources;
- The solicitation of mutually supportive relationships;
- The continuous evaluation for signs that reinforce the selected goals and a determination to endure.

Verifying the attributes

Morse verified these attributes by applying them to other situations where the concept 'hope' was thought to be important. Interviews were undertaken to gauge the experiences of an appropriate sample of patients who were: waiting for a heart transplant, rehabilitating after a spinal cord injury, surviving breast cancer and planning to continue breast feeding. She points out that, if the attributes from the previous phase do not hold true for these new situations, then the analyst must return to the first phase and select another exemplar. If the attributes do hold, then the additional information obtained from the qualitative interviews contributes to the concept analysis.

Identifying manifestations of the concept

While the attributes may be seen in each of the interviewees' experiences, they may not be in the same order or pattern. These variations should be identified. In Morse's (1995) example she noted that the attributes were present in each of the four groups of patients but they were manifested differently. By examining these differences Morse was able to further develop the concept of 'hope'.

2 If the literature review notes that the concept is similar to another, undertake concept delineation

Within nursing there are many concepts that are similar to other concepts: fear-anxiety, comfort-care, etc. Morse suggests that when this occurs a literature review must be done to separate the two concepts in terms of meaning, attributes, and differences and commonalties. She did this for the two concepts 'suffering' and 'enduring'. Interviews were undertaken with patients who were seriously burned and yet who had remained conscious throughout the experience. It became clear from the qualitative data collected that while 'enduring was a state that existed without emotion and focused on the present, suffering was an emotional response to a lost past or an irrevocably altered future' (Morse, 1995: 40). Those who were suffering were very expressive in their grief, while those who were enduring had a 'mask-like' expression.

3 If the literature review suggests numerous concepts to denote one phenomenon, undertake concept comparison

When there are many competing concepts to explain a relatively underdeveloped phenomenon these concepts should be identified and a literature review undertaken. The attributes for each competing concept should be identified, described and compared. The limitations of each concept in explaining the phenomenon should be stated.

Morse (1995) recognised that the concepts 'intuition', 'inference' and 'emotional empathy' are all used to explain the phenomenon of an expert nurse being able to sense the patient's condition with access to very limited data. She compared these three concepts by asking questions related to preconditions, process and outcomes. Preconditions included questions such as: Is it a special talent? Is it learned from the nurse's past? Can the experience be taught? Process questions included: Is the nurse's response emotional, cognitive or physical? At what level of consciousness does the process occur? Outcome questions were: Is the experience accurate in predicting the patient's condition? Is the experience positive or negative for patient care? The answers to these questions indicated that, apart from some overlap, each of the three concepts was unique. None of the concepts accurately explained what was happening when used alone. The concept comparison exercise identified the need for further research into this important phenomenon.

4 If, owing to too much literature on the topic, the concept appears confusing, undertake concept clarification

Morse noted that the concept caring appeared to be well described in the literature. However, on closer inspection she found that the wealth of material left the concept 'murky'.

Once more she recommends a literature review and the identification, description and comparison of the attributes of the concept. The following questions were asked: Is caring unique to nursing? Does the caring intent vary between patients? Can caring be reduced to behavioural tasks? Does the outcome of caring affect the patient, the nurse or both? The answers to these questions allowed the literature to be sorted according to underlying assumptions revealing five manifestations of caring. These were: caring as a human trait, caring as an emotion, caring as a moral imperative, caring as a mutual endeavour and caring as a therapeutic intervention. This process of concept clarification has added considerably to understanding the concept of caring.

5 If the concept within the literature does not adequately explain the phenomenon, undertake concept correction

It may be noted that the concept as it is discussed in the literature does not do justice to the clinical phenomenon it is supposed to represent. In this case, interviews and observations are undertaken in the clinical setting and the data are examined for commonalties and differences between them and the concept that purports to represent them.

Morse (1995) undertook concept correction on 'therapeutic empathy' and noted that it did not fit all the nursing situations in which it was being used. It was found that while nurses used sympathy, pity, compassion and consolation, some of these were discouraged in communication courses in favour of therapeutic empathy. Therefore, Morse noted a discrepancy between the concept taught and those that the practitioners found useful in delivering care.

6 If data exist for which there is no appropriate concept in the literature, undertake concept identification

Compared to other mature disciplines, nursing has come a long way in a short period of time. However, there are still gaps in our conceptual base. With concept identification the nurse may detect what he or she believes to be a new clinical phenomenon. He or she may label it with a conceptual term. He or she will then search the literature to establish that the concept is unique. He or she will identify its attributes, establish if it is present in other contexts and explore its relationship to other related concepts.

Morse invented the concept 'compathy' to explain a portion of data from a qualitative study she was undertaking. It refers to the phenomenon whereby a person feels another's pain. In other words, one person's pain triggers a pain response in an observer. She followed the concept identification process and found that 'compathy' did fill a conceptual gap in the literature.

The six different approaches to concept analysis which Morse (1995) describes represent a departure from the stepwise approach adopted by most other authors. In essence, Morse used qualitative data from real-life situations, incidents and events in an inductive way as a basis for expanding the nursing conceptual base.

Validity and reliability of concept analysis

Validity and reliability of concept analysis are issues which Chinn and Kramer (1995) address. A conceptual analysis is valid if it is based upon multiple examples that are fully representative of the range of meanings of the concept. Reliability may be claimed if the concept can be consistently recognised using the attributes and indicators that you have created.

The criteria of reliability and validity can also be applied to the empirical indicators. The empirical indicators must represent or measure the concept they are supposed to (validity) and they must do so consistently (reliability). Face validity is a little better than no validity and means that, on the face of it, the empirical indicator looks as if it represents the concept of interest. Content validity is a more robust test and is best achieved by asking a panel of experts if they believe that the empirical indicators adequately operationalise the concept.

Theories change over time and, likewise, the attributes of a concept may alter from one period to another. Similarly, depending on their theoretical perspective, different analyses of the same concept carried out by different people may produce different attributes. Therefore, concept analysis, while worthwhile, is often a tentative business; this applies regardless of whether the process is qualitative or quantitative or an admixture of both.

The development of propositions

Although the importance of propositions was referred to in Chapter 1, it is proposed to explore them in greater depth here. To recap, theories are made up of statements about relationships between concepts written in the form of propositions. Therefore, a natural progression from concept analysis and clarification is the building of propositions. According to Meleis (1991), the development of propositional statements is a major step in the generation of theories. There are different types of proposition. Fawcett and Downs (1992) illustrate their usefulness to nursing by dividing them into sets: non-relational (concerning only one concept) or relational (relationship between two or more concepts).

Non-relational propositions

This set of propositions is composed of two types:

Existence propositions: this type of proposition is simply a statement concerning the existence of a concept, e.g., post-operative pain. Existence propositions are important in the development of descriptive theory.

Definitional propositions: these propositions can be:

- Theoretical definitions (a dictionary definition, e.g., pain is 'discomfort or suffering');
- operational definitions (a precise researchable definition, e.g., 'pain exists when the patients states it does');
- empirical indicators (an instrument used to measure the concept, e.g., the presence or absence of pain is indicated by the score on a pain-assessment tool).

Definitional propositions are useful in research reports in that they provide the reader with an understanding of the concepts being studied. However, such propositions limit themselves to the generation of statements that are concerned with only that concept. In other words, the relationship of that concept to one or more other concepts is not described or discussed.

Relational propositions

Relational propositions are the statements of relationship between two or more concepts. They extend the understanding of a concept by showing how it is linked to other concepts. The more developed relational propositions are, the more they are able to define, explain, and predict the nature of the relationship between concepts.

Fawcett and Downs (1992) identify the following relational propositions. Many of the examples used are hypothetical. The concepts are represented by x and y.

- *Existence of a relationship*: this is the most basic of the relational propositions. It merely states that there is a relationship between x and y. It may, for instance, be stated that there is a relationship between self-care and age.
- *Direction of a relationship*: the direction of the relationship may be a positive (direct) or a negative one (indirect) between x and y. For example, providing appropriately focused information to pre-operative patients is positively related to post-operative wellness.
- *Shape of a relationship*: this informs us if there is a linear or curvilinear relationship between x and y. For instance, an increase in anxiety is associated with an increase in cardiac output – here the relationship is linear.
- *Strength of a relationship*: this statement focuses on the magnitude of the relationship between x and y. For example, there is a strong relationship between twelve-hour nursing shifts and low nurse morale.
- *Symmetry of a relationship*: here a relationship between x and y is either symmetrical or asymmetrical.

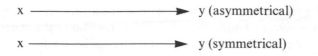

A statement asserting the positive relationship between self-care and knowledge and vice versa is a symmetrical proposition.

- *Concurrent relationships*: this refers to the simultaneous occurrence of x and y – if x occurs then so does y. Fawcett and Downs (1992) provide the example of a concurrent association between functional status and psychological state.
- *Sequential relationships*: the lapse of time between the occurrence of x and y is what is important for sequential propositions. So, if x occurs, then later y will occur. For example, there is a sequential relationship between relaxation therapy and reduced anxiety.
- *Deterministic relationships*: these propositions are concerned with the degree of certainty that something will happen in a particular situation. Therefore, if x occurs, then y will always occur, assuming no change in conditions.
- *Probalistic (stochastic) relationships*: these relationship statements centre on the probability that if x occurs than y will probably also occur. If a nurse teaches a patient how to inject insulin, then the patient will probably gain the knowledge needed to self-administer insulin.
- *Necessary relationships*: these prepositional statements declare that if x occurs, and only if x occurs, then y will occur. The first concept (x) must be present in order for the other concept (y) to present itself.
- *Substitutional relationships*: here, one concept x^1 may be substituted by x^2 and y will still occur. Therefore if x^1, but also if x^2, then y. For example, both lack of sleep and poor nutritional state are related to poor response to therapy.
- *Sufficient relationships*: this type of propositional statement asserts that, if x occurs, a certain other concept, y, will also occur, regardless of anything else. Once more, the example of pre-operative teaching having a positive effect on post-operative recovery illustrates this proposition.

- *Contingent relationships*: here, the occurrence of a relationship between concept x and concept y is contingent on the presence of a third concept, z. For example, the strength of a relationship between pre-operative teaching and post-operative well-being depends on the experience of the nurse practitioner.

Assumptions, research questions and hypotheses

Because assumptions are also statements of relationship between concepts, they are special types of proposition (see Chapter 1). Assumptions are statements which the nurse accepts as true or takes for granted. For example, that humans live in a constantly changing environment is an assumption. As nurses reflect on the concepts and the numerous types of proposition outlined above they may identify explicit and implicit assumptions. Taking heed of their own perceptions, values and beliefs will help in the formulation of assumptions. Assumptions are central components of a theory. For instance, both Roy (1971) and Orem (1980) have eight assumptions underpinning their theories.

Hypotheses and research questions are propositions stated in testable forms. Moody (1990: 175) states that the purpose of generating propositions after the analysis and operationalisation of concepts is to 'facilitate the formation of researchable questions and hypotheses. The subsequent research is also more likely to advance understanding of the concept under study.' The research approach adopted may be qualitative or quantitative in nature.

Research questions and hypotheses are derived from propositional statements by linking each of the concepts in the proposition to their identified empirical indicator (see Step 9 above). By being testable the research questions and hypotheses are connecting the concepts and propositions to science. For example, if a nurse made a statement of a negative relationship between expressing sexuality and urinary incontinence this is a directional proposition. The nurse may convert this into a testable hypothesis by stating that, 'the greater the problem with urinary incontinence the lower the score obtained on Norbert Expressing Sexuality Scale'. Alternatively, a research question could be formulated: Does urinary incontinence have a negative effect on expressing sexuality as measured by the Norbert Expressing Sexuality Scale? Research may then be undertaken (and hopefully replicated) to obtain results which will answer the research question, or support or refute the hypothesis. Whether supportive or not, the findings will help in the development of new theoretical knowledge. If supportive, the nursing care undertaken with patients who have urinary incontinence will be altered to take account of the problems such patients may have with expressing their sexuality.

In conclusion, readers will note that a phenomenon occurring in the clinical area can provide nurses with hunches that will lead to the identification of a concept. This concept may be analysed qualitatively or quantitatively (or through a mixture of both) in order to clarify its meanings. The relationship between this concept and other concepts can be made explicit by formulating propositions. These propositions may be converted into research questions or hypotheses which, when addressed through research, will provide new theoretical knowledge and new practices.

Summary

Concept analysis is an important process in a developing discipline such as nursing. There are many reasons for this, not least that concepts are the building blocks of theories and, if their characteristics are not well developed, problems of understanding and meaning will result in confusion and conceptual disarray. Most of the methods of concept analysis emanate from Wilson's (1969) work and entail a series of steps. More recently, Morse (1995) denigrates this as reductionism and suggests a more qualitative approach to concept analysis. The reader should examine both and decide which of these approaches fits the concept of interest and their purpose in undertaking the analysis. There are many types of proposition and these can grow out of the clarification of concepts. Hypotheses and research questions developed from propositions can be addressed by research studies. Therefore, theorising commences in practice and returns to inform practice.

The additional reading section at the end of this chapter gives an overview of several concepts that have undergone analysis in the literature.

Additional reading on concept analysis

Araklian, M. (1980) 'An assessment and nursing application of the concept of locus of control', *Advances in Nursing Science*, 3: 25–41.

Ashmore, R. and Ramsamy, S. (1993) 'The concept of the "gaze" in mental health nursing', *Senior Nurse*, 13: 46–9.

Beyea, S.C. (1990) 'Concept analysis of feeling: a human response pattern', *Nursing Diagnosis*, 1(3): 97–101.

Boyd, C. (1985) 'Towards an understanding of mother–daughter identification using concept analysis', *Advances in Nursing Science*, 7(3): 78–86.

Brownell, M.J. (1984) 'The concept of crisis: its utility for nursing', *Advances in Nursing Science*, 5: 51–88.

Crawford, G. (1982) 'The concept of pattern in nursing: conceptualised development and measurement', *Advances in Nursing Science*, 5: 1–6.

Davis, G. (1992) 'The meaning of pain management: a concept analysis', *Advances in Nursing Science*, 15(1): 77–86.

Forsyth, G.L. (1979) 'Analysis of the concept of empathy: illustration of one approach', *Advances in Nursing Science*, 2: 32–42.

Green, J.A. (1979) 'Science, nursing and nursing science: a conceptual analysis', *Advances in Nursing Science*, 2: 57–64.

Haase, J.E., Britt, T., Coward, D.D., Leidy, N.K. and Penn, P.E. (1992) 'Simultaneous concept analysis of spiritual perspective, hope, acceptance and self transcendence', *Image: The Journal of Nurse Scholarship*, 24: 141–7.

Henneman, E.A., Lee J.L. and Cohen, J.I. (1995) 'Collaboration: a concept analysis', *Journal of Advanced Nursing*, 21: 75–82.

Jacob, S.R. (1993) 'An analysis of the concept of grief', *Journal of Advanced Nursing*, 18: 1787–94.

Knafl, K.A. and Deatrick, J.A. (1986) 'How families manage chronic conditions: an analysis of the concept of normalisation', *Research in Nursing & Health*, 9: 215–22.

Knafl, K.A. and Deatrick, J.A. (1990) 'Family management style: concept analysis and development', *Journal of Paediatric Nursing*, 5(1): 4–14.

Kolcaba, K.Y. (1991) 'A taxonomic structure for the concept comfort', *Image: The Journal of Nurse Scholarship*, 23(4): 237–40.

Mairis, E.D. (1994) 'Concept clarification in professional practice: dignity', *Journal of Advanced Nursing*, 19: 947–53.

Meeberg, G.A. (1993) 'Quality of life: a concept analysis', *Journal of Advanced Nursing*, 18: 32–8.

Meize-Grochowski, R.M. (1984) 'An analysis of the concept of trust', *Journal of Advanced Nursing*, 9: 563–72.

Newberry, V.B. and Krowchuk, H.V. (1994) 'Failure to thrive in elderly people: a conceptual analysis', *Journal of Advanced Nursing*, 19: 840–9.

Norris, C.M. (1975) 'Restlessness: a nursing phenomenon in search of meaning', *Nursing Outlook*, 23: 103–7.

Olsen, R.S. (1985) 'Normalisation: a concept analysis', *Rehabilitation Nursing*, 10: 22–30.

Panzarine, S. (1985) 'Coping: conceptual and methodological issues', *Advances in Nursing Science*, 7: 49–57.

Pless, B.S. and Clayton, G.M. (1993) 'Clarifying the concept of critical thinking in nursing', *Journal of Nurse Education*, 32: 425–8.

Rawnsley, M. (1980) 'The concept of privacy', *Advances in Nursing Science*, 2(2): 25–32.

Reckling, J.B. (1994) 'Conceptual analysis of rights using a philosophical approach', *Image: The Journal of Nursing Scholarship*, 26: 309–14.

Rew, L. (1986) 'Institution: concept analysis of a group phenomenon', *Advances in Nursing Science*, 8(2): 21–8.

Simmons, S.J. (1989) 'Health: a concept analysis', *International Journal of Nursing Studies*, 26(2): 155–61.

Slevin, E. (1995) 'A concept analysis of, and proposed new term for, challenging behaviour', *Journal of Advanced Nursing*, 21: 928–34.

Stephenson, C. (1991) 'The concept of hope revisited for nursing', *Journal of Advanced Nursing*, 16: 1456–60.

Teasdale, K. (1989) 'The concept of reassurance in nursing', *Journal of Advanced Nursing*, 14: 444–50.

Teel, C.S. (1991) 'Chronic sorrow: analysis of a concept', *Journal of Advanced Nursing*, 16: 1311–19.

Trandel-Korenchuk, D.M. (1986) 'Concept development in nursing research', *Nursing Administration Quarterly*, 11: 1–9.

Ward, C. (1986) 'The meaning of role strain', *Advances in Nursing Science*, 8(2): 39–49.

Watson, S.J. (1991) 'An analysis of the concept of experience', *Journal of Advanced Nursing*, 16: 1117–21.

Whitley, G.G. (1992) 'Concept analysis of fear', *Nursing Diagnosis*, 3(4): 155–61.

Chapter 4
Introduction to nursing theories

This chapter will examine in depth the theoretical journey that nursing has made and is still making. It will explore how our practice, research, education and theorising have been influenced both positively and negatively by theories from other disciplines. Particular emphasis will be placed upon the advantages and limitations of those grand theories that are perceived to be the property of nursing.

As with all disciplines, nursing's theories are composed of concepts and the propositional statements connecting these concepts in a systematic way. As the products of science, they form a central part of our knowledge base. However, for most of the twentieth century nursing has been dominated by a wide array of theories from other disciplines. Perhaps the one that has had the most effect has been the medical model.

The medical model

Florence Nightingale (1859) was of the opinion that medicine and nursing should be clearly differentiated from each other, and during her time this was indeed the case. Prior to the establishment of her nurse training school at St Thomas's Hospital in London, nurses were lower-order figures who were the 'handywomen' of the community. They were often paid for their services with gin, and to make their calls they often had to walk the streets alone at night, something a respectable woman would never do. In contrast, physicians came from the respectable middle and upper-middle classes and invariably their social and educational backgrounds were very different from those of the nurses who took orders from them.

Therefore, prior to Nightingale's interest in reforming nursing, it has to be said that there already existed a differentiation between these occupations. This is probably not the type of differentiation Nightingale meant. She did not believe that doctors cured; rather that nature or a healthy environment was responsible for the curing. At the end of her book *Notes on Nursing* she argues:

> It is said that medicine is a curative process. It is no such thing; medicine is the surgery of functions, as surgery is that of limbs and organs. Neither can do anything but remove obstructions; neither can cure; nature alone cures. Surgery removes the bullet out of the limb, which is the obstruction to cure, but nature heals the wound. So it is with medicine; the function of an organ becomes obstructed; medicine, as far as we know, assists nature to remove the obstruction, but does nothing more.

Nurses could be actively involved in this process of 'putting the patient in the best condition for nature to act upon him' if given appropriate training. This may also remove them from their subservient position to the physician. Nightingale stated that, 'if I have succeeded in any measure in . . . showing what true nursing is, and what it is not, my object will have been answered.'

However, Nightingale often contradicted herself. Although she is quoted as saying that obedience was 'suitable praise for a horse' (Woodham-Smith, 1977), her nursing schools encouraged obedience to the doctor. Further, the influences she derived from religion (use of the terms 'sister', 'vocation') and the military (hierarchy, duty and the idea of a uniform) also brought with them the requirement of unquestioned obedience. To lend support to this interpretation of Nightingale's influence, Wood (1880), a contemporary of Nightingale, stated that, 'In the training of nurses we should aim at making them intelligent, conscientious hand-maidens to the medical staff.'

It was unfortunate that Nightingale's intense interest in research and its methods was not passed on through her nurse training courses. In contrast, medical students, who were mostly male, studied in universities where they were taught the importance of scientific enquiry and publication. The social order of the day did not assist in the development of a knowledge base for nursing. Expertise in Latin was essential to gain entrance to medical school and Latin was a language not normally taught to women (Peplau, 1987).

Therefore, in the nineteenth century Nightingale's desire for a differentiation between doctors and nurses was realised: they were separated by their gender, social class, language and education. This differentiation was to remain for most of the twentieth century. Meave stated that:

> Nurses are wounded healers who can be very hard to live with. Many of us are burned out, oppressed, unhappy, demeaned, and victimised, making it difficult not to actualize these feelings in our practice. Much of this angst can be laid at the feet of medicine.
>
>   (Meave, 1994: 14)

If nurses were to assist doctors, then it was important that they were well prepared for this role. In the 1970s doctors were still being asked to lecture to nurses about nursing, and textbooks written by doctors were required reading on psychiatric and general nursing courses. Peplau (1987) argues that those who teach control the content of an occupation. Through such brainwashing, nurses inherited a slavish adherence to a Cartesian reductionist philosophy where human beings were often seen as the sum of their parts. The medical perspective also inculcated within nurses' minds ideas that illnesses were caused by genetic, biochemical, traumatic or pathological disturbances, and could be treated by the physician using medications or surgery.

The scientific basis for the medical model can be traced back to Hippocrates, Aristotle and Galen. In the early seventeenth century Descartes fostered the notion of the body as a machine (see Chapter 2), of disease as the consequence of breakdown and of the physician's task as repair of the machine. Wright (1986) argued that being subservient to medicine was at the genesis of nursing's rigid adherence to task-centred care.

The treatment of McMurphy, the patient in *One Flew over the Cuckoo's Nest* (Kesey, 1962), is an example of this reductionism. McMurphy was perceived as a malfunctioning machine and nursing duties were split into medication rounds, bath times, meal times. There was a tendency to view staff as observers and patients as the observed. In this situation, things, people and events are broken down into their constituent parts. There is some evidence that this process is also dominant in other institutionalised services such as prisons, religious orders and the army (see Goffman, 1961).

Most physicians base their treatment philosophy on the fundamental tenet of reductionism. This implies that all behavioural phenomena must be conceptualised in terms of physiochemical principles (Engel, 1977). Over the years this basic precept has been accepted, not only by many health care professionals but also by the public.

Engel (1977) believed that physicians' attitudes are moulded by the medical model long before they embark on their professional training. It is incorporated within the human socialisation process. Medical education reinforces this early indoctrination with its emphasis on the structure and function of the body and the integrity of anatomical parts and physiological systems.

This reductionist view appears to ignore the many social and psychological influences to which individuals are susceptible (Engel, 1977). However, in some instances these influences are taken into account, albeit in a subordinate relationship to physical changes in the person. Medical education focuses on the physical sciences of biology, physics, chemistry, histology and pathology. Little time is given to the study of sociology, psychology and philosophy. Therefore, the main emphasis of the medical model is on the nature side of the nature–nurture continuum.

Within the medical model, the preliminary assessment is of great importance to physicians. The initial examination will ultimately lead to the recognition of signs and symptoms. Kim (1983) believes that proponents of the medical model have a vested interest in searching for abnormal clinical features to confirm the presence of illness. These signs and symptoms are categorised into patterns which, in turn, form the basis for diagnostic labelling. Chapman (1985) maintains that such labelling has a dehumanising effect because the client is envisaged as little more than a disease entity.

For the medical model, knowing the disease inevitably determines the treatment strategy. The goals of therapy are seldom client-centred and the individual must assume the client role with the concomitant obligation to co-operate (McKenna, 1990). This compliance is an important element in the treatment process. There is also a perception that nurses will comply and co-operate with the physician's orders. Nurses are discouraged from providing information to the patient about their possible prognosis – this is the doctor's job and the desire to meet goals within a nursing care plan is not a sufficient reason for a patient to remain in care once the medical treatment is complete. Therefore, while the therapeutic plan may present the facade of the egalitarian team approach, the doctor, as the healer, is viewed as superior to all other disciplines (Mitchell, 1986).

Nursing and the medical model

Because of the traditional hierarchy within health care, nurses were subservient within a handmaiden role (Aggleton and Chalmers, 1986). This servile position is seen by many to be due to tenacious reliance on the medical model (McFarlane, 1986b; Meave, 1994). According to Peplau,

> Well into the 1940s, many textbooks for nurses, often written by physicians, clergy, or psychologists reminded nurses that theory was too much for them, that nurses did not need to think but rather merely to follow rules, be obedient, be compassionate, do their duty, and carry out medical orders.
>
> (Peplau, 1987: 18)

According to Stockwell (1985), as an observer of signs and symptoms, the nurse is the eyes and ears of the doctor, and as a practitioner the nurse is his or her hands and feet, carrying out the prescribed treatment. Such a focus does not allow for independent action, and a danger exists that it may lead practitioners to ignore aspects of the client which do not fit neatly within the boundaries of the medical model. Contained within this framework of treatment, nurses may be ill-equipped to help the client as a whole person.

The constraints of the medical model affect care in other ways: Stevens (1979) wondered if our adherence to a medical philosophy has not influenced our choice of the nursing process. She noted that its essential components bear more than just a passing resemblance to the problem-solving approach used in medicine. More recently, George (1995: 3) argued that the nursing process has its basis in the positivist approach to science. This, in itself, may not be damaging to our profession, but Baldwin (1983) noted that within the 'process' practitioners tended to use medical terms to define goals of care. Ward staff frequently use the language of symptoms to describe client behaviours, and classify clients into diagnostic types. For example, rather than nurses assessing the patient's problem as 'chronic bronchitis', a medical term, they should focus on the problems concerning the effect that chronic bronchitis is having on the patient and his or her family. These may include problems with sleeping, eating, walking, communicating, etc.

Because of intense scrutiny, the limitations of the medical model have become more apparent. Paramount among these is the philosophy of the 'sick role'. Parsons (1952) recognised that clients, as exemplified by the sick role, have the right to be relieved from social roles and the right not to be held responsible for their illness or condition. They are, however, obliged to seek professional help and to try their best to get well. This nurtures the 'pill for every ill' sentiment where individuals, if experiencing anxiety, tension or low mood, are viewed as ill, and such problems are considered appropriate targets for drug treatment (McKenna, 1990). This strategy diverts attention away from potentially important social and psychological factors, which have little currency within the medical model. That one person differs from another in terms of race, sex, age, marital status, religion or social class is given merely the briefest consideration.

Our adherence to physicians' orders has fostered a fascination with cure, with the possibility of care being placed in a secondary position. Like our medical colleagues, many nurses have shown preferences for work in acute settings where discharge is expected and so-called technical skills are given high status. The long-stay wards and units for care of the elderly are less popular choices and tend to be staffed by large numbers of untrained personnel.

Although the medical approach to modern nursing is increasingly queried (Huch, 1995), there is evidence that it still remains a major influence in the delivery of care (Stevens-Barnum, 1994). Junior doctors' hours are being reduced and many of their technical duties are being transferred to nurses. In turn, nurses may transfer much of their 'basic nursing care' to untrained assistants. Another word for 'basic' is 'fundamental', and some of these delegated activities are the very foundations of caring. Nurses must ensure that slavishly following the medical agenda does not leave them in a type of 'limbo' between caring and curing. Like social work and occupational therapy, the nursing profession is in a state of flux, trying to decide whether to relate to, or seek independence from, physicians.

The medical model does have major advantages for the treatment of illness. Advances in medically oriented cures have freed many clients from the effects of disturbing symptomatology and contributed to their early discharge. Many nurses have gained life-long employment as a result of adopting a medicalised view of health care. Mitchell (1986) outlines yet another contribution: he believes that because of its universality, prospective clients are familiar with it and as a result the public find it comforting to be cared for within a framework they can recognise.

It is important that practitioners take cognisance of these factors and realise the imprudence of rejecting the medical model in its entirety. Within any nursing theory, the biological and pathological perspective of the individual must be acknowledged. None the less, nursing's disenchantment with the pervasiveness of the medical model has been one of the main reasons for the development of theories in nursing.

Nursing theories

Walker and Avant (1995) identify four levels of theory. These, in part, reflect Merton's (1968) categorisations (see Chapter 1).

- Metatheory
- Grand theory
- Mid-range theory
- Practice theory

Metatheory

Nursing theory has become an important part of our discipline and is in equal partnership with nursing research and nursing practice. As the number of theorists have increased so have the number of 'theory watchers'. These individuals are called metatheorists and, while they do not formulate theory themselves, they discuss, debate, describe, analyse, categorise, classify and explain what theorists are developing and how practitioners and patients are affected by such developments. In essence, they develop theories about theories. They form a growing and important body of scholarly watchdogs who are not beyond adding a critiquing role to their many other duties.

Metatheorists include but are not limited to Meleis (1991), Stevens-Barnum (1994), Walker and Avant (1995), Fawcett (1995), Kim (1983), Marriner-Tomey (1994), George (1995), and Dickoff and James (1968). Another role for these metatheorists is to examine how changes in the various philosophies of science affect the change in emphasis among nursing theorists. To some extent, therefore, metatheory incorporates the examination of how theory affects and is affected by research and practice within nursing, and philosophy and politics outside nursing. They have a powerful voice in shaping the future of nurse theorising. To some, metatheorists are frustrated theorists: they can tell their readers how to generate, apply and test theory, but there is no evidence they can do it themselves. However, Meleis (1995) has developed a theory of transitions and Parse (1995) has taken on a metatheorist role in some of her writings.

In Chapter 2, I referred to Dickoff and James's 'theory of theories'. The following brief description will serve to illustrate this key metatheoretical work. I will be returning to their work throughout this book as an exemplar of metatheory. They published a series of papers in 1968 identifying four theoretical levels within nursing. These were:

Factor-isolating theory: theories at this level are sometimes referred to as 'naming theories' because they name, describe and classify concepts. The end result of this level of theorising is descriptive theory.

Factor-relating theory: theories at this level seek to explain phenomena by relating named concepts to one another. The product is explanatory theory.

Situation-relating theory: theories at this level seek to anticipate relationships among concepts or propositions. The result of theorising at this level is predictive theory.

Situation-producing theory: theories at this level seek to assign actions which lead to specific outcomes. The end result of such theorising is prescriptive theory.

Dickoff and James (1968) maintain that a higher level of theory cannot be generated until theory at the preceding level has been formulated. They reason that, since nursing is a practice discipline, the goal should be to have theory at this fourth level. Such theories would enable us to prescribe nursing interventions which had a positive effect on patient well-being.

Through their 'theory of theories' Dickoff and James indicated that theory can exist at different levels of abstraction, and even the naming of concepts could be perceived as theorising. Their work caused much debate and set the agenda for practice-related nursing theories. As metatheorists, Dickoff and James influenced nurse theorists in how they should develop their work. They also influenced other metatheorists, such as Meleis (1991) and Stevens-Barnum (1994), to adopt the belief that models and theories were synonymous (see Chapter 1).

Grand theory

In Chapter 1 the differences between nursing theories and nursing models were discussed and the designation 'grand theory' was suggested as an alternative term to 'model'. As we enter the twenty-first century, nurse theorists have formulated over fifty grand theories of nursing. Furthermore, there are many borrowed theories which have been used successfully by nurses to influence practice, and more mid-range and practice theories are being formulated each year. Some of the grand theories have been developed inductively, from experiences in practice; deductively, from other theories (both borrowed and home grown); or through a retroductive combination of induction and deduction. Twelve of the grand theories that exist are British in origin, while most of the rest are from the North American region. However, it was not always like this.

Historical perspective

Nightingale (1859) probably never saw herself as a theorist, but by studying *Notes on Nursing* and the wealth of correspondence she has left us, we recognise with hindsight that she held strong views on health and nursing care. Applying the metaparadigm to her writings, nurse historians noted that she recognised the importance of the individual–environment relationship as a prerequisite for health. She is therefore credited with laying the foundations for nursing's development as a science (Chinn and Kramer, 1995). Her influence on modern theorists who also focused on the person–environment link is clear (Rogers, 1980).

There occurred at the turn of the century some isolated instances of nurses attempting to conceptualise (Norris, 1970). However, these efforts were pre-empted by the adoption of the medical model, which was to permeate nursing education and practice (see above). The resultant theoretical hiatus within nursing persisted until the 1950s, leaving us with almost a 100-year period within which there was little evidence of explicit theorising in nursing. There are several reasons for the renewal of interest in the mid-twentieth century:

- Disagreement with the medical model as a proper focus for our discipline (Farmer, 1986);
- The desire to develop a scientific basis for our practice (Aggleton and Chalmers, 1987);
- The contribution of women to the Second World War effort (Chinn and Kramer, 1995);
- The perceived importance of actively involving clients in their own care (Rambo, 1984);
- The advent of university education for nurses (Meleis, 1991);

- The increase in the number of master's/doctoral dissertations prepared by nurses (Hardy, 1978);
- The quest for professional recognition (Fawcett, 1995).

Hildegard Peplau (1952) has been given credit for formulating the first contemporary theory in nursing. She developed her theory both inductively, through reflecting on a long career in psychiatric nursing, and deductively, through the influence of the interpersonal theory of Henry Stack Sullivan (1953). Peplau's work greatly influenced later theorists who used 'interpersonal relationships' as a basis for their work (i.e., Henderson (in Henderson and Harmer), 1955; Orem, 1959; Johnson, 1959; Hall, 1959). These early efforts were largely concerned with identifying concepts, and many historians within the discipline refer to these pioneers as the 'conceptualists' (Meleis, 1991). The resultant theories were often developed to underpin curriculum content rather than practice or research – a pattern which was to repeat itself much later on this side of the Atlantic.

Nurse theorising thrived in the early 1950s on the courses taught at Columbia University's Teachers' College, where the influence of the philosopher and staff member John Dewey permeated the curricula. Dewey (1933) emphasised the practical application of knowledge, focusing particularly on how philosophical and theoretical thinking can work in everyday life. To the pragmatist Dewey, truth was something that worked in practical experience and had to be adaptive to needs and circumstances. Columbia Teachers' College was the Alma Mater of theorists such as Peplau, Henderson, Hall, King, Wiedenbach and Rogers. Abdellah's doctoral dissertation was prepared there under the supervision of Peplau (see Meleis, 1991).

The publication of the first issue of the journal *Nursing Research* in 1952 provided a forum for theorists and researchers to debate the development and testing of theory by rigorous and systematic enquiry. None the less, according to George (1995), these early theorists operated from the perspective of the medical model, focusing mainly on *what* nurses did rather than how or why they did it.

The 1960s saw the publication of theories by Abdellah *et al.* (1960), Orlando (1961), Wiedenbach (1964), Levine (1966)

Travelbee (1966) and King (1968). Of these theorists, Abdellah, Orlando and Travelbee were undoubtedly influenced by Peplau's earlier work. During this period, the development of theories was given an added impetus by an increase in journal articles and conferences on various aspects of theorising (Suppe and Jacox, 1985).

In 1965, the American Nurses Association stated that theory development was one of the most significant goals for the profession. This facilitated the widespread interest in conceptualising which pervaded the American nursing services of the 1960s. As a result, nursing theory became the framework for structuring many nurse training programmes, leading to the unwelcome possibility that theory would be synonymous with education rather than practice. Also in the 1960s, the US government made funds available for doctoral study for nurses. This funding fostered the development of future nursing theories and theorists.

In the mid-1960s, Henderson, Wiedenbach and Orlando, previously students at Columbia, all gained employment as lecturers in Yale School of Nursing. Here, theorists began to study how nurses practised and the effect this had on patients. Myra Levine, while also working at Yale, put forward her 'conservational' theory of nursing (Levine, 1966). It was also at Yale that the philosophers Dickoff and James (1968) wrote their seminal work on a 'theory of theories', which led nurses to realise that they, as practitioners, could make a major contribution to the formulation and use of theory.

The attempts to theorise in the 1960s led to a desire to define what nursing was, as evidenced by the now famous 1966 definition of nursing by Henderson. This trend of definition searching had the potential to cause confusion among practitioners. Could the unique definitions of fifteen nurse theorists all be correct? Furthermore, having explicit definitions for nursing tended to create boundaries and discouraged a search for knowledge outside these boundaries.

The rapid growth in the number of nursing theories in the 1960s continued into the 1970s, with the work of Roy (1970), Rogers (1970), Neuman (1972), Riehl (1974), Adam (1975), Patterson and Zderad (1976), Leininger (1978), Watson (1979) and Newman (1979). Unfortunately, there was little in the way of critique and analysis. Many of the theorists simply stated their theory and made no effort to explicate propositions in the form of theoretical assumptions. Theorists were praised at conferences and honoured with doctorates from universities. Few nurses wanted to be accused of anti-intellectualism by openly debunking the new theories. The lack of empirical testing of these theories meant that 'the emperor had no clothes', but not many were willing to say so publicly.

In 1972, the National League of Nursing specified an accreditation criterion emphasising that curricula should be based upon a theory (Meleis, 1991). This was followed by the formation of the Nursing Theories Conference Group (1975) and the Nursing Theory Think-tank (1979), both formed to assist practitioners to use theories in order to guide their clinical work. Several interesting publications and discussion papers emanated from these bodies (George, 1975, 1985).

While the 1980s witnessed an acceptance of the significance of theories for the discipline, in America at least, there seems to be a slowing down in the number of grand theories being developed. In the US, only three new nursing theories were published in the 1980s: the work of Parse (1981), Fitzpatrick (1982) and Erickson, Tomlin and Swain (1983).

It seemed that in previous decades nurses were searching for theoretical tools while in the 1980s they decided to sharpen and polish these tools. As a result, many of the theorists began revising their work and examining how mid-range theory could be formulated deductively from their grand theory. This movement will be discussed in detail below.

In the 1960s and 1970s several theorists were reluctant to claim theoretical status for their work. They used the terms 'model' or 'conceptual framework'. Such reluctance was not as evident in the 1980s and 1990s. For example, in her 1968 publication, King outlined her 'conceptual frame of reference' while in her 1971 book, she appeared to be heading 'towards a theory of nursing' which, when revised in 1981, revealed her 'theory of nursing'. This theoretical momentum is also evident in the writings of other theorists (Watson 1979, 1985). Interestingly, metatheorists also seemed to be using the term 'theory' more freely in the 1980s than they had done in the past.

There was another significant development in the early 1980s. New theorists such as Parse (1981) and Fitzpatrick (1982) built their work on Martha Rogers's earlier theory (1970). This 'borrowing' of theory from other nurse theorists represents a new and interesting departure for the development of nursing knowledge.

In the 1990s scholars began to elaborate on the previous work of nurse theorists, updating its meaning for the twenty-first century. For instance, Forchuk (1991) expanded Peplau's theory, making it more amenable to research and practice. Also in the 1990s Boykin and Schoenhofer published their theory of caring. This made a considerable contribution to the previous theories of caring put forward by Madeline Leininger (1978), Jean Watson (1979) and Simone Roach (1984). Furthermore, Rogers (1990), Newman (1994), Neuman (1995) and Parse (1995) updated their theories.

In addition, many nurses in the 1990s have access to the Internet and are able to network, discuss and debate theoretical issues on electronic communication lists devoted to the work of Orem, Parse, Rogers and Erickson, *et al.* There is also a World-Wide Web site devoted entirely to nursing theories. New generations of nurse theorists are publishing their work, and many of the pioneer nurse theorists of the 1950s and 1960s have died: Martha Rogers died in 1994, Virginia Henderson and Myra Levine died in 1996.

The 1990s saw a new surge of energy being focused on theorising in nursing. A new journal, *Nursing Science Quarterly*, edited by Parse, featured articles solely aimed at theory development and testing. A resurgence of interest also occurred in Europe. In 1996 the first European Nursing Theory Conference was held in Malmo in Sweden; the second is being held in Frankfurt in 1997. Also in 1996, metatheorists such as Meleis and Kikuchi presented keynote addresses at theory conferences in the United Kingdom.

Nurse theorising in the United Kingdom

Although Florence Nightingale (1859) formulated her nursing concepts in mid-nineteenth-century England, the United Kingdom does not boast a pedigree of theory development. It appeared that British nurses were content to adhere to Nightingale's teachings on religion, obedience and her pledge to assist the physician in his work, rather than her tenacious commitment to research and science.

In the 1980s and 1990s, some British nurses followed their American counterparts and began to formulate theories. One can include in this the work of Roper, Logan and Tierney (1990), McFarlane (1982), Stockwell (1985), Wright (1986), Castledine (1986), Clark (1986), Minshull, Ross and Turner (1986), Green (1988), Bogdanovic (1989), Friend (1990), Yoo (1991), and Kirby and Slevin (1995). You will note that when there was a slowing down in the development of new theories in the US there was a surge in theory development in the UK.

The stimulus for these theories may have been the perception that American theories were not suitable for practice in the UK. Further, the introduction in the UK of higher education for nurses in the late 1970s forced many lecturers and students to look at how knowledge unique to these disciplines might be developed on this side of the Atlantic. A similar trend can be seen in other countries of Europe and in Australia, where nursing programmes are being delivered within tertiary education. As happened previously with their American counterparts, UK nurses began to examine the medical model and found it an inappropriate framework for viewing nursing and those individuals who require nursing care.

The classification of grand theories

Comte (see Chapter 2) identified several positivist sciences, all of which used taxonomies to categorise those elements which were central to their discipline: botanists classify plants; chemists classify gases; biologists classify cells; sociologists classify groups; and astronomers classify planets. Since the mid-1970s, nurses continued this positivist trait. Since they wished to be seen as belonging to a scientific discipline, various attempts were made to categorise the large number of grand theories. This grouping of theories by various attributes can lead to an understanding of the many paradigms and schools of thought that underpin each theory. Assignment to a category is arbitrary and, while categories are often mutually exclusive in the natural sciences, this is not often the case in nursing.

Perhaps one of the most enduring methods of categorising theories is to allocate them to one or more of the broader 'world view' paradigms (systems, interactional, developmental and behavioural) alluded to in Chapter 1. Occasionally, a system of cataloguing theories arises when the editor of a book tries to arrange them into some orderly scheme. For example, Meleis (1985) organised theories into: those that describe what we do, those that describe how we do it, and those that describe the why of practice. In contrast, Stevens (1979) used the following classifications: 'intervention', 'conservation', 'substitution', 'sustenance' and 'enhancement'. Marriner-Tomey (1994) sorted theories into: 'humanistic', 'interpersonal', 'systems' and 'energy'. Parse (1987) categorised theories under the 'simultaneity' and 'totality' paradigms. Because Parse's classification system is currently leading to much debate in the literature (Cody, 1995), it will be described in detail.

The simultaneity and totality paradigms of nursing

Rosemary Parse (1987) reminds us that a scientific discipline like nursing encompasses more than one paradigm with which to guide practice and research. Each paradigm, or world view, gives rise to several theories. The theories reflect the belief and value system of the parent paradigm so that the concepts and propositions within a theory are congruent with the views set forth in the paradigm. Therefore, the development of science occurs within the context of paradigms (Parse, 1987: 3). According to Parse, nursing science has developed and continues to develop within two almost contradictory paradigms. These are the totality and simultaneity paradigms. More recently, William Cody (1995), a Parsean scholar, has argued that these two paradigms are unique to nursing. He also argues that all aspects of nursing knowledge can be categorised into one or other of these paradigms.

The *totality paradigm* sees the person as an organism whose nature is a composite of bio-psycho-social and spiritual dimensions. The environment is the internal and external stimuli surrounding the person. The person has to manipulate and interact with the environment in order to achieve goals and to maintain health, which is viewed as a dynamic state of bio-psycho-social-spiritual integrity and balance. The goals of nursing focus on health promotion, care and cure of the sick and the prevention of illness, while those receiving nursing care are people who are viewed as ill by society (Parse, 1987: 32).

The totality paradigm has been, and on the authority of Parse continues to be, the predominant paradigm in nursing. It has its roots in the mechanistic Newtonian and Cartesian views of science and dovetails completely with the philosophy inherent within the medical model. This paradigm has given rise to theories that have guided research, education and practice in nursing. The resultant theories tend to centre on helping the sick individual to adapt, undertake self-care, interact and attain health. Within these conceptualisations, the authority figure and prime decision maker is the nurse. Nursing practice is guided by a linear nursing process approach whereby the patient's problems are assessed, a plan of care is drawn up, interventions are undertaken and the results are evaluated. The totality paradigm gives rise to research which is quantitative in nature and where causal and associative relationships are testable.

Moody (1990) states that the work of the following theorists is based within the totality paradigm: Nightingale (1859), Johnson (1959), Leininger (1978), Levine (1966), Neuman (1982), Roy (1971), Orem (1985) and King (1981). One would suspect that many of these theorists would be angry at being grouped under the 'totality' umbrella. They may not have intended in their theories to give the impression that a person is no more than the sum of their parts nor that they had been influenced consciously or otherwise by the medical model.

In contrast, the *simultaneity paradigm* is a more radical view of the world of nursing. It was first propounded by Martha Rogers (1970) and elaborated upon by Parse (1981). The simultaneity paradigm differs from the totality paradigm in three significant ways:

● In its assumptions about the person and health;
● In relation to the goal of nursing;
● In the implications for research and practice.

Within the simultaneity paradigm the person is viewed as a unitary being who is in continuous mutual and simultaneous interaction with the environment. People are viewed as different from, and more than, the sum of their parts. They give meaning to situations and, as 'open beings', are responsible for choices in moving beyond what exists at present (Parse, 1981). Health is viewed as a 'process of becoming' and as a set of value priorities. Health is experienced by the individual and therefore can only be described by that individual. There is no optimum health: health is how one experiences personal living.

The goals of nursing centre on quality of life from the person's perspective. The perception of illness in terms of social norms is not a significant issue within the simultaneity paradigm. According to Parse (1987: 136, 137), nursing illuminates meaning and focuses on the movement of the person and family 'beyond the moment relative to changing health patterns'. There are no care plans constructed around health problems. The prime decision maker and authority figure is the patient, not the nurse. In essence, the patient determines the activities for changing health patterns; the nurse 'in true presence with the person' guides the way. Moody (1990) identifies Rogers (1970), Newman (1979) and Parse (1981) as the theorists whose work best fits the simultaneity paradigm.

Research approaches within this paradigm are mainly qualitative in nature. In 1987, Parse believed that such a methodological approach was a start and stressed that new methods more suitable to the simultaneity paradigm would be forthcoming. In her 1995 book, *Illuminations,* she describes a research approach which is more in keeping with the simultaneity philosophy.

In Chapter 2, the idea of science through revolution put forward by Thomas Kuhn (1970) was described. He proposed that a discipline goes through a period of normal science where one paradigm reigns supreme. This period ends in 'crisis' when the accepted paradigm fails to account for new phenomena that may have arisen as a result of social change or scientific discovery. A revolution then occurs and a new paradigm becomes the accepted way of viewing research, theory and practice. Currently, the simultaneity paradigm is gaining in recognition and increasingly is being used to guide research, education and practice. Perhaps we are witnessing a Kuhnian shift from the totality paradigm to the simultaneity paradigm, and those nursing theories belonging to the former will soon be relegated to the archive of nursing's past knowledge base.

Limitations of grand nursing theories

In the three decades from the 1950s to the 1970s there seemed to be a reluctance to criticise the work of nurse theorists. Perhaps the main reason for this was that most nurses had not the theoretical and philosophical knowledge base necessary to mount a coherent critique. The hero worship that existed for the major theorists may also have been a reason why few critics wanted to be 'out of step' with the masses. There is still evidence of such hero worship: a glance through the Parse, Rogers or Erickson *et al.* lists on the Internet will show that these theorists still have their adoring disciples. Similarly, a view of the many conference videos available of nurse theorists gives another glimpse of the hero worship. In their defence, though, there is no evidence that theorists view themselves as heroes. None the less, in the 1980s and 1990s grand theories in nursing underwent a degree of criticism and their many disadvantages were highlighted.

Webb (1986a) differentiates between low-level and high-level criticisms, the former being more easily overcome than the latei.

The low-level criticisms can be summarised as follows:

1   *Too many theories*: At last count there were approximately fifty grand nursing theories and several dozen mid-range theories. It would be almost impossible for hard-pressed clinicians to be *au fait* with all these theories, nor, according to Clark (1986), should they be so.

2   *Jargon*: most of the available theories are characterised by esoteric language. This has been referred to as 'abstract jargon' (Wright, 1985), 'verbal diarrhoea' (Houlihan, 1986) and 'semantic confusion' (Hardy, 1986). This is seen as contributing to the unmanageability of theories in practice. There is also the danger that the use of this 'jargonese' will lead to widespread confusion, not only among practising nurses but also among the public and our multidisciplinary colleagues (McFarlane, 1986a).

'Parsimony' dictates that all theories should be elegant in their simplicity (Walker and Avant, 1995). This is often referred to as 'Occam's razor', after Sir William of Occam who, in the twelfth century, argued that man (*sic*) should seek the simplest explanation for a phenomenon. In other words, a good theory is stated in the simplest terms possible. Therefore, the theorist has a responsibility to put forward a point of view which people can understand.

Unfortunately, most nursing theories have paid little attention to the concept of parsimony. For example, although Rogers (1970) is quoted as emphasising the need to avoid jargon, her theory views the environment as 'a four dimensional nega-trophic energy field identified by pattern and organisation, and encompassing all that is outside any given human field'. Stevens (1979) stated that Rogers may be held in high esteem by those nurses who assume that any theory must have merit if they cannot understand it, in other words, those who believe a good theory is one you cannot understand!

The language usage within other theories is just as problematic and may lead to confusion. For example, 'adaptation' in one theory (Roy, 1971) is taken to mean something totally different from 'adaptation' in another theory (Levine, 1966). Similarly, a 'stressor' is viewed as a negative stimulus in one theory (Roy, 1971), while it is defined as a positive force in another (Neuman and Young, 1972).

The obtuseness of jargon could not be discussed without giving an example of the terminology from Rosemary Parse's theory: 'The practice methodology emerges directly from the ontology, and with the human becoming theory, structuring meaning multidimensionally, co-creating rhythmical patterns, and cotranscending with possibles lead to the practice processes of illuminating meaning through explicating, synchronizing rhythms through dwelling with, and mobilizing transcendence through moving beyond' (Parse, 1993: 12).

Although acknowledging the overuse of jargon in theories, Aggleton and Chalmers (1987) believe its identification as a major criticism is 'unduly cynical'. Theory must have complexity in order to be significant. After all, since the concepts under study are abstract, precise theoretical language must, of necessity, be complex (Duldt and Griffin, 1985). The problem is not only unique to theories within our discipline: Freud's (1949) theory introduced the terms 'ego', 'superego', 'id', 'Oedipus complex', 'Electra complex', etc. Furthermore, in the example from Parse, the reader should remember that Parse was heavily influenced by Heideggerian phenomenology and her use of words demonstrates that she has remained true to this philosophy of science.

Webb (1986b) believed that practitioners have a professional obligation to make an effort to understand the vernacular of theories. After all, she points out, the learning of any new subject, be it music, law or gardening, requires that the student become familiar with a new language. A nurse may be willing to learn new medical terms when it suits the occasion, but may also berate the use of new nursing terms even though they may improve care by giving the nurse a new perspective from which to view clinical phenomena.

3   *Documentation*: the emphasis on increased paperwork when using theories has alienated many practitioners. For many nurses, the implementation of theories is seen as a 'paper exercise'. This view is hardly surprising considering that Miller (1985) found that Roy's theory required sixteen A4 pages for its proper application. But perhaps we should not blame the theory for this; it is but a tool, and we can decide how to use it.

McKenna found in his 1992 study that practitioners were able to inform him as to which nursing theory they applied to practice. This tended to reflect the documentation they were using. However, he noted that, while the documentation may have been based upon a recognised explicit theory, the care being delivered was not. Staff did not have a 'mind-set' for the theory and the theory did not appear to cross the threshold of the ward office.

4   *The suitability of American theories*: as outlined above, the large majority of nursing theories have their origin in the United States, and people have questioned how far these theories are transferable to practice in Britain. Wright (1986) suggests that

there is nothing wrong with professionals from different nations swapping ideas, but that the application of one group's practices to the other may not always be appropriate. Therefore, if British nurses continually look towards America for conceptual guidance, a manipulative process will have to be employed to assure the validity of US theories within the British health service. Furthermore, nursing theories from the United States have their roots in a different culture, a different health care structure and a different nurse education scheme.

This problem is not isolated to the United Kingdom. Other European nurses are writing about nursing theories (Hunink, 1995) and theories of nursing are being developed on the European mainland. Examples of these include van Bergen and Holland's (1980) self-reliance/self-realisation theory and van den Brink-Tjebbe's (1985) self-care theory. The latter references and more information on these Dutch nursing theories can be found in Arets and Slevin (1995).

5 *Staffing issues*: Chavasse (1987) recognises the importance of high staffing levels when attempting to use theories in practice. She believes that if a theory identifies goals that cannot be met due to lack of time, the staff are likely to become extremely frustrated. This may also raise ethical issues. One wonders if it is morally right to uncover multiple nursing problems with a client when, because of staff shortages or short lengths of stay or the predominance of the medical model, only a few of these problems will be addressed. There is also the argument that in a ward where individualised client care is practised, there will be different staffing requirements than in a ward that practises the 'block treatment' method of task-oriented care.

The high-level criticisms are summarised below:

1 *Conceptual substance*: Fawcett (1995) states that most of the grand theories currently available in nursing are all-embracing, abstract, non-testable conceptual models. Therefore, in an attempt to be all-inclusive, nursing theories explain nothing. This belief that theories are general statements about care has led some to the idea that a theory can be utilised in a wide

range of settings. This blanket application of one theory may, according to Hardy (1986), be unwise and even dangerous.

There is also the contrary condemnation which states that these same grand theories have adopted a restricted view of nursing because theorists have trodden a narrow path in their efforts to theorise (Webb, 1986a). In the discussion above, the medical model has been castigated for its emphasis on reductionism. However, Webb (1986a) argued that the theories of Roper *et al.*, Roy, Henderson, King and Orem *reduce* the client to a list of activities, needs, modes of adapting or to a set of self-care requirements.

2 *Ideal concepts versus practical reality*: the majority of theories deal with practice as it ought to be, and not as it is. Meleis (1991), in considering this problem, felt that theorists were becoming more competent in articulating what theory is, rather than what the substance of practice itself is. It is argued that, if we do not know what nursing is, how can we work within the real world of practice? However, if grand theories merely reflect the status quo in nursing, then their implementation in a clinical area would not herald any significant change in how nurses practise. Further, if much current practice is still based on the medical model, as some suggest (Stevens-Barnum, 1994), then grand theories reflecting the real world of nursing will be supporting continued adherence to the medical frame of reference. Minshull *et al.* (1986) intimate that this is happening. They state that Roper, Logan and Tierney's (1990) activity of living theory is 75 per cent medically oriented.

Therefore, perhaps theories should focus on how nursing ought to be. However, this also leads to problems: those who wish to introduce a theory into the clinical setting may be met by sceptical practitioners who see theories as merely the results of academic exercises aimed at increasing the complexities of their lives. Within the UK, nursing theories have taken over the unpopular position recently vacated by the nursing process.

Nurses are often characterised as being anti-intellectual when it comes to research, higher degrees and the nursing process

(Webb, 1986a). This anti-scholarly attitude also extends to theories. Although the apparent divorce between what theorists believe and what goes on in the busy clinical situation is one reason for this, the imposition of theories by management encourages similar reactions. This introduction by force of a theory that calls for individual choice is an obvious contradiction.

Benefits of grand nursing theories

Those who advocate the use of theories outline a number of advantages thus gained. Two distinct benefits have already been discussed. These are the substitution of nursing theories for the medical model, and the conviction that theories lead to the development and expansion of nursing knowledge. These are without doubt important gains both for clients and professionals. However, the literature highlights several other equally favourable contributions of nursing theories.

1   *A guide for practice*: it has been argued that the implementation of the nursing process without a theory to underpin it is an empty approach, often described as 'practising in the dark' (Aggleton and Chalmers, 1986). Although European nurses have only recently been introduced to theories, they have been wrestling with the nursing process for some time. Wright (1986) asserted that they got the cart before the horse. By providing a systematic basis for assessment, planning, implementation and evaluation, theories are seen to offer a way to 'revitalise' the nursing process.

    Therefore, in order to be implemented successfully and to have meaning for practitioners, the nursing process as a problem-solving approach must be framed within a nursing theory. As a supplement to this role, nursing theories also stress the importance of the wholeness and integrity of the person, thus further enhancing the practitioner's ability to provide individualised care. Being templates for the provision of care, theories are essential guides for action and, as such, they help bring theoretical knowledge and clinical practice closer together.

    The usefulness of these frameworks has also been recognised

in the areas of nursing education (Rambo, 1984), administration (Fawcett, 1989) and research (Nicholl, 1992).

2   *Education*: although the dichotomy between classroom and ward is well documented (Meleis, 1991; Chambers, 1995), there is evidence to suggest that the structuring of an education pro- gramme around a theory is extremely beneficial for students (Aggleton and Chalmers, 1987) and, as a result, theory and practice may eventually meet. Grand theories do at least attempt to identify what nursing is, who the recipients of nurs- ing care are and what skills and knowledge bases practitioners should possess. Therefore, they can be perceived as adding sound structure to curricula.

   A study, using a thirteen-item Likert-type scale with sixty- nine subjects from the same nursing school, found that the students' practice was positively influenced by their use and knowledge of a nursing theory (Hagemeire and Hunt, 1979). Jacobson (1987) undertook research in the US to describe how nurses regard theories. The research subjects, graduate nursing students and their teachers, were presented with a forty-three- item questionnaire. Most of the respondents (76 per cent) were enthusiastic about nursing theories. When asked how impor- tant nursing theories were for the advancement of nursing, most of the students and staff believed them to be 'crucial'.

   In 1991 Salanders and Dietz-Omar reported the results of an American survey into whether nurses believed that nursing theories helped them in clinical decision making. Data were collected at three points in time: before taking a nursing theory course, on completion of the course and two years later. Data collected at both post-course points indicated that, according to respondents, 'nursing theories did indeed provide a frame of reference for clinical decision making'.

   More recently, McKenna (1994b) compared the attitudes of university-based and college of nursing-based student nurses. Both groups of students were positive in their regard for nurs- ing theories with the college students being significantly more positive than the university students. All respondents believed that theories lead to better individualised quality of care.

3   *Professionalisation*: the use of theory as a basis for practice is one of the characteristics of a profession. Smith (1986) maintains that nursing could achieve full professional status comparable with other professions by basing its practice on theories. Theories are also seen as harbingers of autonomy and responsibility, leading to professional accountability, and they assist nurses in describing and explaining what they do and in predicting outcomes from nursing interventions (Meleis, 1991). Furthermore, by having their roots in phenomena which are of specific importance for nurses, nursing theories help to differentiate nursing from other disciplines. The professionalisation of nursing through the use of theories may also ensure us a place as equal colleagues in the multidisciplinary team. Smith (1982: 118) argues that the use of nursing theories helps to make explicit to other professional groups that there is something called nursing which has an identity of its own, distinct from other similar activities. This would be a tremendous leap forward in the development of nursing as a profession.

4   *Quality of care*: in one study, McKenna (1994a) found that the quality of care given by a practitioner using a theory is high because practice is built on a systematic knowledge base. He found statistically significant improvement in the processes and outcomes of care as a result of theory being used. There are other strong indications that nurses must practise from a theoretical foundation if care is to be of good quality. George (1995) re-emphasised this view, asserting that quality of care can only improve when the foundations for that care are supported by theories. Similarly, the quality of a service cannot be assessed unless there are standards against which an appraisal can be made. Farmer (1986) asserts that the setting of standards requires the adoption of a theory. To support this, Goodridge and Hack (1996) stated that theory-based practice may significantly affect nursing care quality through influencing standards of practice.

    Quality of care evaluation in contemporary practice is becoming increasingly related to cost-effectiveness. If used appropriately, nursing theories can demonstrate cost-effectiveness through reducing dependency, reducing nursing's preoccupation with non-nursing tasks, encouraging client self-care, and the early detection of clients' problems (Webb, 1986a). Nursing theories can also assist in bringing about desired patient outcomes (Sorrentino, 1991). In addition, using a theory to underpin practice allows staff a greater articulation of health goals, hence identifying more efficiently the resources and skills needed to achieve them.

Boxes 4.1 and 4.2 summarise the major contributions and criticisms of nursing theories. While these statements have been garnered from the literature, most are opinions rather than evidence from research studies. As a result some are contradictory.

Box 4.1 Perceived contributions of nursing theories

- Assist student learning (Gordon, 1984);
- Help to structure patient assessment (Webb, 1986a);
- Permit meaningful communication between nurses (McFarlane, 1986a);
- Improve problem solving (Gottlieb and Rowat, 1987);
- Increase patient satisfaction (Hoch, 1987);
- Identify the goals of practice (Jennings and Meleis, 1988);
- Substantially improve quality of care (Fawcett and Carino, 1989);
- Clarify nurses' realm of accountability (Fawcett, 1989);
- Focus observations on important phenomena (Schmieding, 1990);
- Guide and justify nursing actions (Firlit, 1990);
- Clarify thinking among nurses about practice (Kershaw, 1990);
- Provide others with a rationale for nurses' work (Barber, 1986);
- Direct research towards clinical nursing needs (Girot, 1990).

Box 4.2 Perceived criticisms of nursing theories

- Do not prepare nurses for the reality of practice (Hardy, 1982);
- Offer little guidance for nursing action (Webb, 1984);
- Too abstract, academic, idealistic and irrelevant (Miller, 1985);
- Are not responsible for any change in practice (Sternberg, 1986);
- Lead to premature closure on ideas (Kristjanson, Tamblyn and Kuypers, 1987);
- Their application is a criticism of current practice (Luker, 1988);
- Provide only the illusion of positive change (Luker, 1988);
- Mislead practitioners because they do not describe reality (Botha, 1989);
- Provide only tentative ideas about practice (Chalmers, 1989);
- Are unable to cope with multiple clinical foci (Kemp, 1990);
- Are not empirically tested or evaluated in practice (Walsh, 1990).

Mid-range theory

Like concepts, theories may be classified by their levels of abstraction along a continuum from grand theories to practice theories. As alluded to above, grand theories are broad and abstract and do not easily lend themselves to application or testing. In contrast, narrow-range theories are very precise and restricted in their focus. Moody (1990) argues that for a theory to be usefully generalised to other nursing situations, it needs to be abstract. But this means that it is difficult to operationalise the concepts within a theory and, without measurable indicators, how can the concepts and propositions be tested through systematic and rigorous research?

Mid-range theories go some way towards solving this problem. They are moderately abstract and inclusive but are composed of concepts and propositions which are measurable. Therefore, mid-range theories, at their best, balance the need for precision with the need to be sufficiently abstract. First advocated by the sociologist Robert Merton (1968), mid-range theories are more focused than grand theories. They have fewer concepts and variables within their structure, are presented in a more testable form, have a more limited scope and have a stronger relationship with research and practice.

Merton (1968) maintained that mid-range theories were particularly important for practice disciplines. He stated that they identify a few key variables, present clear propositions, have limited scope and can easily lead to the derivation of testable hypotheses. They may be developed deductively and retroductively, but more often they tend to be developed inductively, using qualitative studies.

Walker and Avant (1995) maintain that mid-range theories balance this specificity with the conceptual economy normally seen in grand theories. As a result, mid-range theories provide nurses with the 'best of both worlds' – easy applicability in practice and enough abstract ideas to be interesting scientifically. Although their work has only recently received increasing attention in the UK, American metatheorists were calling for the development of mid-range theories concerning the management of pain and the promotion of sleep over twenty years ago (Jacox, 1974).

Like branches of a plant that grow out of control, mid-range theories can sprout in all directions, leading to fragmentation of the discipline's knowledge base. However, in the 1990s, nursing has recognised the phenomena that specifically interest us, the importance of the metaparadigm, and the grand theories that help identify the boundaries of our discipline. As a result, Meleis (1991) believes that the time is right for the development of mid-range theories.

Mid-range theory deals with a relatively broad scope of phenomena but does not cover the full range of phenomena that are of concern within a discipline. A theory of pain alleviation represents a mid-range theory for nursing; it is broader than a theory of neural conduction of pain stimuli but narrower than the goal of achieving high-level wellness. The phenomenon of pain is a mid-range concept of concern for nursing because it is only one of many phenomena that comprise the global concern of the discipline (Chinn and Kramer, 1995: 216).

Mid-range theory tends to focus on concepts of interest to nurses. As well as pain, these include empathy, grief, self-esteem, hope, comfort, dignity, quality of life. Mid-range theory can also grow from concept analysis (see Chapter 3) and is inextricably linked to research and practice. This triad of research–theory–practice helps to close both the theory–practice and the research–practice gaps and to provide knowledge which is more readily applicable in direct care situations.

Some mid-range theories have their basis in grand theories. For example, the mid-range theory of 'self-care deficit' grew out of Orem's (1980) grand theory of 'self-care'. This supports Smith's (1994) assertion that a major function of grand theories is to act as a source for mid-range theory development. By doing so, they ensure that the focus of mid-range theories remains a nursing one. Fawcett (cited in Smith 1994) agrees, believing that, if a 'conceptual framework' (*sic*) is not related to mid-range theory, then it is not absent but is really present in an implicit sense. However, other mid-range theories grow directly from practice. For example, Swanson's (1991) mid-range theory of 'caring in perinatal nursing' was inductively developed from studies in three perinatal settings. Similarly, Mishel (1990) developed a mid-range theory of 'uncertainty' among patients.

Chinn and Kramer (1995) discuss eight other mid-range theories which can be used to guide practice. These include a theory of menstrual care, a theory of family care-giving, a theory of relapse among ex-smokers, a theory of uncertainty in illness, a theory of the perimenopausal process, a theory of self-transcendence, a theory of personal risk and a theory of illness trajectory.

Practice theory

According to Jacox (1974), the development of mid-range theory seems particularly well suited as a basis for the development of practice theory. Practice theories are normally very specific in their clinical focus and they are narrower in scope and more concrete in their level of abstraction than mid-range theories. Jacox (1994: 10) defines 'practice theory' as 'a theory that says given this nursing goal [producing some desired change or effect in the patient's condition], these are the actions the nurse must take to meet the goal [produce the change]'.

Ten years earlier, Wald and Leonard (1964) were the first to argue for a 'practice theory' to guide nursing actions. They maintained that theory should emanate from practice, be used and tested in practice, and have incorporated within it causal hypotheses. In other words, with practice theory a nurse should be able to say 'if I do this, then the following will happen'. Therefore, practice theory prescribes the clinical interventions of the practising nurse.

Glaser and Strauss (1967) identified the grounded theory approach to developing theory and reasoned that a good theory should provide specific guidelines for prescribing practice. The following year Dickoff and James (1968) (see above) identified four levels of theory. They urged nurses to aim for the highest level, 'situation-producing theory'. Theory of this type provides practising nurses with prescriptive guidelines for action leading nurses to undertake appropriate interventions. They stated that the major contention is that theory exists for the sake of practice (because, in a sense, every lower level of theory exists for the next highest level and the highest level exists for practice), and that nursing theory must be theory at the highest level (because either the nursing aim is practice or else nursing is no longer a profession distinct from a mere academic discipline) (Dickoff and James, 1968: 101).

This view of practice theory as a directive for action is criticised by Lorraine Walker (1971: 429) who sees this as an 'odd use of the term theory'. She states that normally the term 'theory' is employed in the context of systematic description and explanation rather than prescription. Jacox (1974) disagrees, stating that in a practice discipline like nursing, theory is not just something that describes and explains; theory specifies that given the need to produce some change in the patient's condition these are the actions that the nurse must undertake. For instance, nurses know that they can reduce the patient's experience of pain by undertaking specific actions and that the possibility of pressure area damage can be reduced by regular turning. Similarly, to reduce the possibility of post-operative anxiety, the nurse knows that providing the patient with information before surgery will ensure that he or she will experience less anxiety after surgery. Because this may not happen every time with every patient it is not a law; however, since it should have the desired effect with most patients it is practice theory. By using practice theory, the nurse is going further than simply describing, explaining or predicting a phenomenon.

Walker's criticism of Dickoff and James's ideas was not seen as a particularly valid one. Later, Beckstrand (1980) put forward a more substantial criticism, arguing that nursing does not need specific 'practice theories' because existing scientific and ethical theories already provide us with the information we require for successful nursing interventions. This criticism has been countered by Gray and Forsstrom (1992), who are thankful that not all nursing authors take Beckstrand's perspective. Their counter-argument centres on the need for nursing as a distinct discipline to have specific theoretical underpinnings for its actions. More recently, Walker and Avant (1995: 12) point out that they see little difference between what some nurses do normally in their everyday 'practice' and 'practice theory'. They suggest that some people may wish to 'drop the word theory . . . and think of practice theory as nursing practices'.

It must be acknowledged that, since Dickoff and James's fourth level of theory (see above) aims at prescription (control), it is heavily influenced by the positivistic view of science. This charge is further supported by their view of theory development being a hierarchical one where level four is infinitely better for nursing than level one. In fact, it could be argued that if practice theory is founded on cause-and-effect thinking then randomised controlled trials and experimental designs generally are the designs that most nurses would have to use. Qualitative designs, by their very nature, have difficulty in establishing relevant cause-and-effect associations. This statement would bring renewed criticism from those who favour the historicist philosophy of science. Should nurses be concerned with such criticisms? A pragmatist such as Larry Laudan (1977) would say, 'who cares, so long as the generated theories identify interventions that solve clinical problems'. More will be said about pragmatism in Chapter 5.

Practice theory is undergoing a revival, with the focus on practitioners reflecting from practice and formulating theory which will return to inform practice. Wooldridge (1992) maintains that:

- Practice theory should be stated in such a way that the assumed cause–effect relationship between the mean(s) and the goal(s) can be empirically tested.
- Practice theory should focus on causal agencies that are manipulable by the practitioner, on effects that are deemed relevant to evaluating the achievement of practice goals, and on those contingent conditions that are applicable to practice situations.
- Practice theories developed by a given profession should focus on means for which that profession can assume autonomous prescriptive authority, both through direct manipulation of practice and through the structuring of practice guidelines.

The current emphasis on the development of clinical guidelines in the United Kingdom could be construed as a 'practice theory' generation process. Clinical guidelines are research-based protocols for best practice. Staff at centres in York, Leeds, Liverpool and Oxford undertake comprehensive world-wide reviews of research studies on particular clinical topics. From these reviews they design guidelines for best practice. Since these guidelines specify what actions should be taken to achieve specific outcomes, they may be referred to as 'practice theories'.

Much confusion still exists on the differences between mid-range and practice theories. For example, Hall (1993) referred to Parse's theory as a practice theory. Parse (1993) disagreed, asserting that this gives the impression that the theory comes empirically from practice, whereas she sees her work as the frame of reference to guide practice. She views her theory as the science of nursing and the application of her theory to practice using specific methods as the art of nursing.

The role of reflection in the development of practice theory

The view of practice theory put forward by Dickoff and James (1968) clearly focuses on the prescription of interventions so that specific outcomes will be achieved. According to Diers (1979), the most appropriate research method to obtain theory at this level is

the experimental approach. However, another way of defining practice theory is as any theory which grows out of clinical practices,
experiences and activities. Kim (1994), for instance, sees practice
theory as that which underlies a nurse's understanding of a clinical
situation or event and the decisions she or he makes with regard to
that situation or event. The preferred method for formulating this
type of practice theory is reflection. This view of practice theory,
and the methods used to generate it, differs significantly from that
of Dickoff and James (1968), Jacox (1974) and Wooldridge (1992).

As a process, reflection is undertaken in order to gain understanding, insight and new knowledge about practice. Because of
this it is often called 'praxis' (Brent, 1993). Glaser and Strauss
(1967) maintain that working to gain insight is the source of all significant theorising. Therefore, obtaining insight through reflection
is a core activity in formulating theory. Reflection can enable us to
make sense of our clinical work by mapping out a pathway through
the 'swampy lowlands' of practice.

Chinn and Kramer (1995: 218) recognise the important role that
reflection plays in 'personal knowing'. They define reflection as 'an
inner process that requires integrating a wide range of perceptions in
order to realise what is known within the self'. They identify three
stages: 'engaging', 'intuiting' and 'envisioning'. 'Engaging' simply
means the direct involvement of the nurse in the situation.
'Intuiting' is the subjective perspective the nurse brings to the situation based upon his or her previous experiences. 'Envisioning'
occurs when the nurse's creative intuition gives a unique meaning to
the situation and reveals new possibilities. During these stages the
nurse may reflect on possible answers to questions such as: Why
did that happen? Why did the patient respond like that? How did I
know exactly what to do? Could this be the reason?

A broader view of reflection was taken by Boud, Keogh and
Walker (1985). They stated that reflection is more than just idle
daydreaming, rather it is perusal with intent, a purposive activity
directed towards some goal. They also identify a series of stages in
the reflective process. These are:

● recollection of experience;
● attending to own feelings;

- re-evaluating the experience through
  association,
  integration,
  validation,
  appropriation.

In order to facilitate reflection it is recommended that a detailed record is kept of the situation or event. This may be done through the use of logs, journals, diaries or debriefing sessions with colleagues. Gray and Forsstrom (1992) used this process to develop practice theory. They found that the recollection of experience occurs as the diary is being written.

The second stage identified by Boud and colleagues involves not just describing the situation perceived but actually taking cognisance of one's own feelings towards the situation. Old entrenched beliefs should not be allowed to influence the perception. When possible, these should be replaced with an openness and a fresh way of viewing the experience. Once more, this can be achieved as the diary is being written.

Stage three of Boud *et al.*'s reflective process is composed of four parts. The first part, 'association', enables the reflective practitioner to connect what they have experienced during the situation with their pre-existing knowledge and actions. The end result may be that the individual substitutes old attitudes or knowledge with new learning. An effective way to achieve this is to have a brainstorming group where all ideas and perceptions are open to discussion; this helps clarify thoughts and feelings and leads to new insights. Brainstorming groups also help generalise the new insights where they are applicable to other individuals and similar situations that group members may have encountered.

The next step in Boud *et al.*'s process of reflection is 'integration'. Here, the individual begins to discriminate between the many ideas, feelings and issues that arose during association. As a result of this discrimination, relationships may be identified and conclusions may be reached. New concepts, beginning propositions and assumptions may also be uncovered. Furthermore, it may be possible to see linkages with existing theory.

'Validation' involves comparing our new insights with the

experiences, knowledge and insights of other practitioners to note the authenticity of our feelings. In this way we see if our new awareness is reliable and valid. Validation also entails trying out our new way of viewing things in different situations. Gray and Forsstrom (1992) feel that, within nursing, the best method of validation is to take the new insights back to the clinical area and test them there.

Appropriation is the final step in Boud *et al.*'s framework. Essentially, appropriation means incorporating the new attitudes and insights within our revised knowledge base – making them our own. As a result, the new knowledge can be used in future encounters with situations that led to the reflection in the first place. This encourages the link between reflection and action, for without action reflection is an empty process.

Appropriation does not mean that you have reached the end of the process or that future reflection should not take place when faced with similar scenarios. Rather, reflection is an ongoing process – a journey not a destination. The following is an example of reflection using Boud *et al.*'s framework.

Recollection of experience

As part of a larger study, I spent nine months collecting research data on two long-stay psychiatric wards (McKenna, 1992). As part of the action research design, I interviewed the patients and staff many times during this period and came to know them very well. About four months into the study, a rumour began circulating that both wards were going to close and that the patients were going to be transferred. The patients and staff were concerned about this and, for a different reason, I too was concerned. Because of my perceived neutrality, patients and staff asked me to approach the hospital managers and find out if there was any truth in the rumours.

The managers assured me that as far as they were concerned there would be no planned closure of any wards in the foreseeable future. I informed the staff and patients of this and the rumours ceased. When the study was completed several months later I left the wards. I was reluctant to leave as I had made many friends on the wards.

About six months later I returned to the hospital to see if the changes made during the action research study had been sustained. I recorded the visits in a personal journal. I was surprised to find that the wards had been closed and were now refurbished as an administration block. The patients and staff had been transferred to several other wards within the hospital. I visited most of these patients and found that many were unhappy on their new wards.

Attending to one's own feelings

I recorded how I felt in the journal, and the best way to describe my feelings was as a mixture of guilt, anger and sadness. Guilt because, based on information I had received, I had assured these patients that their wards were not going to close. I also felt guilty because there was the possibility that deep down they may have thought that my study was, in some way, related to the eventual ward closure. I experienced anger because I felt I had been duped by the system. I felt sadness when I thought that these people's homes had been taken from them without their involvement in the decision-making process.

Re-evaluating the experience

Association: I began my psychiatric nurse training in 1972 and in my *naïveté* I thought that these large hospitals with all their staff and patients were a permanent fixture in health care. Despite my early concerns with institutionalisation, I realised that many patients and staff associated such places with security, caring and permanency. While aware of the political climate and the desire for the community shift, I was still surprised at the closure of the study wards. I revised my feelings and perceptions and was able to associate this event with other recent instances of powerlessness among psychiatric patients (see McKenna, 1994b). As part of my action research study I had set out to empower and involve the patients and staff in decision making. The closure of the wards occurred without any such involvement or empowerment. I was also able to associate what had occurred with previous experiences of how junior nursing staff are treated in general and psychiatric services. Today, many staff are in temporary positions and do not know if or when they will be on day duty, night duty or indeed laid off work completely.

I was able to brainstorm these perceptions and beliefs among a group of mature practitioners who were undertaking a master's degree in nursing at the University of Ulster. This was helpful in that I realised that the experiences and feelings I had were not isolated ones. From these discussions it was possible to generalise many of my feelings of anger, sadness and guilt to other situations.

Integration: as a result of the brainstorming that took place with the students, I was able to discriminate between many of my feelings. The guilt was an unrealistic feeling because the reason for ward closure was a political one, and if there was a guilty party it was probably social policy. While the philosophy underpinning hospital closure is in the main a beneficent one, the use of power and vested interests have led to poor practices. This exercise had the effect of reducing my anger but not the feeling of sadness for the innocent people who had become powerless victims of political and policy decisions.

My conclusions were that, despite the rhetoric about choice and charters, patients and practising nurses are not empowered as they should be and power remains in the hands of managers and policy makers. It struck me that, from a philosophy of science point of view, the critical science approach was the most relevant way of viewing these issues (see Chapter 2). This led to more reflection and the identification of the key concepts of involvement, collaboration, empowerment, valuing, hierarchy and policy. It was possible for me to formulate beginning propositions indicating negative relationships between policy and hierarchy and patient and staff empowerment, involvement and collaboration.

Validation: I returned to the student group to validate my feelings about the loss of power among patients and staff in psychiatric hospitals and to discuss the concepts and beginning propositions uncovered during the integration stage. I also reviewed the literature and newspapers and collected a great deal of information about the powerlessness of ex-psychiatric patients. Yet another method of validation involved gaining access to other psychiatric wards. I was able to do this quite easily in my role as placement tutor for psychiatric nursing students. From many open-ended conversations with patients and staff I found a sense of helplessness and in some instances hopelessness. All this data seemed to confirm the insights I had gained regarding the relationship between power and politics.

Appropriation: as a result of my reflections and the discussion with others I have incorporated this new information within my knowledge base, my teaching and my practice. I also plan to test the beginning propositions using rigorous and systematic research approaches. This forms the basis for a practice theory, in that, by realising the problems related to lack of empowerment, involvement and collaboration, practitioners can plan programmes where these principles are encouraged. The critical science approach of education, enhancement, emancipation and empowerment will provide the philosophical underpinning.

Kemmis (1985) viewed critical science as an appropriate framework for reflection noting the influence that Jurgen Habermas (1971), a founder of critical science, had on the development of reflection. In considering the above example of reflection, Kemmis's opinion is apt: he stated that critical reflection aims at recovering and examining the historical and developmental circumstances which shape our ideas, institutions and modes of action as a basis for formulating more rational ideas, more just institutions and more fulfilling forms of action.

Reflecting on reflection as a basis for practice theory

Practice theory, as a product of reflection, has the advantage that it is based in the real world of clinical nursing. In contrast, grand theories are mostly focused on the ideal world of what nursing could or should be. While practitioners may use reflection, they do not normally perceive themselves as theorists. It is possible that, while some clinical nurses may see themselves as reflective practitioners, they would feel insulted if they were called theorists. To them, theorists are ivory-tower nurses who do not look after real people in real situations.

However, as a process, reflection also has its drawbacks. It is a skill and, like all skills, it must be learned through practice and study. Without these skills reflection may be non-productive at best and may simply undermine the practitioner's confidence and competence at worst. Furthermore, as with the Heideggerian view of phenomenology (see Chapter 2), it may not be possible for individuals during the 'association' stage to put traditional attitudes and beliefs on hold in order to gain new insights. In the above example I do not know if I was successful in ignoring my previous biases and looking at the issues objectively. Alternatively, perhaps the traditional attitudes I held brought an extra dimension to my reflections.

Reflection also heavily relies on memory, and our memory 'playing tricks on us' can lend bias to our reflections (Newell, 1992). Psychological literature also reminds us that anxiety can affect our willingness to recall events and situations. Accepting this, Newell states, we should also question the validity and reliability of the outcome of reflection. None the less, the development and practice of reflective skills, the use of brainstorming groups and the keeping of accurate diaries may go some way towards counteracting these weaknesses.

Theory linkages

In this chapter four main levels of nursing theory have been examined: metatheory, grand theory, mid-range theory and practice theory. It is possible to identify the following connections between these levels. Going down the ladder of abstraction, metatheory clarifies grand theory, grand theory guides mid-range theory and mid-range theory directs practice theory. Going up the ladder of abstraction, practice theory tests mid-range theory in practice, mid-range theory refines grand theory and grand theory provides material for metatheory (Walker and Avant, 1995).

Hunink (1995) differentiates these levels of theory by using the analogy of a map: if a grand theory is envisaged as a map of a country, a mid-range theory is a map of a county within the country and a practice theory is a map of a village within the county. In this analogy, a theorist would be a cartographer and a metatheorist would be a person who studies that cartographer's craft.

Summary

The discipline of nursing has come a long way in a short space of time. Prior to Nightingale, nurses and the clergy looked after people in their own homes and in private institutions. Nightingale gained power and recognition by identifying the fundamental characteristics of good nursing. Unfortunately, modern nursing inherited Nightingale's teachings on obedience and vocationalism rather than her love of enquiry through rigorous research. After Nightingale, nursing was greatly influenced by its adherence to the medical model. This influence was seen by many to be detrimental to the development of a knowledge base unique to nursing. In the 1950s, a group of American nurses began to theorise about nursing. Thirty years later, nurses in the United Kingdom also attempted to isolate theoretically the core of good nursing. There have been numerous taxonomies used to categorise the resultant theories. Although the rationale behind such classification may be viewed as positivist reductionism, it has enabled nurses to study the origins, differences and similarities of these theories.

Grand theories are useful in that they give a broad perspective of the boundaries of our discipline. In recent years there has been an increase in the number of mid-range theories being produced. These theories have their basis in research and practice and are more user-friendly than the highly abstract grand theories. Theories which guide practice were discussed in the theoretical literature of the early 1960s. There has been a resurgence of interest in such practice theories in the 1990s. Some people view them as theories that enable practising nurses to prescribe nursing interventions. Others take a broader focus and see them as knowledge that arises from practice and can return to guide practice. This latter view of practice theories has been encouraged by the current interest in educating nurses to become reflective practitioners.

On both sides of the Atlantic, nursing theories have been lauded by some and attacked by others. The viewpoint adopted in this text is to recognise that debate and disagreements are healthy in a pluralistic discipline like nursing. These theories are simply tools and as such they may be used and then put aside as their usefulness wanes.

Chapter 5

Choosing a theory for practice

The ultimate justification for the existence of theory is to give humans a view of their world which may help them describe, explain or predict events, or prescribe actions which will enable events to occur or not. Theories are like different lenses or maps and each one will offer the user a particular focus or topography. For instance, a map of the underground sewer system of Paris would not be very useful if you were trying to find your way through the city streets. Similarly, a pair of opera glasses would not serve your purpose if you wanted to view the night sky.

According to William Cody (1994) theory is a distinct and well-articulated system of concepts and propositions rooted explicitly in a philosophy of nursing and intended solely to guide nursing practice and research. If we accept this definition then we must be careful in our selection. If we choose the wrong map we may find ourselves at a different destination from the one chosen. Therefore, perhaps a central selection criterion is 'fitness for purpose', in other words, does the theory serve the purpose for which it is intended?

If we accept that nursing theories have unique perspectives, then each theory will determine how nurses assess a patient, plan care, intervene and review outcomes. Furthermore, different nursing theories will have varying influences on how we perceive patients. For instance, one theory may encourage dependence by stressing that the nurse should do everything for the patient, while another may encourage independence by stressing that the nurse should teach the patient about self-care.

Therefore, an unsuitable choice of a theory could easily have detrimental effects on patient care. We must also be careful that the theory chosen does not become an ideology to enslave us. This happens when we forget the aforementioned purpose of describing, explaining and predicting reality and instead accept one theory's view of reality as the only one. When this occurs we consciously or subconsciously create enemies of those who support opposing viewpoints, we diminish the views of others, assert control over our views of truth and deny the presence of other realities (Smith, 1994). As mentioned in the previous chapter, currently in the literature and on the Internet theory lists (http://www.oise.on.ca/~jnorris/nt/theory.html) there is some evidence of this tunnel vision with Parseans, Rogerians or Watsonians worshipping their own particular gospel.

The process of transforming a theory into an ideology may be helped by the imposition of grand theories on busy practitioners. Chapman (1990: 14) describes a typical United Kingdom selection strategy: senior nurses and tutors decide which theory will be used in each ward or unit, and charge nurses and staff are requested to become acquainted with it (with varying amounts of help from the school and service side), and to interpret and use it on their ward. Enthusiasm may understandably be lacking, so the minimum is done to satisfy the requirements.

Gould (1989) observes that it seems unfair that managers or academics, even with the best of intentions, should thrust theories on hard-pressed practising nurses who are facing the reality of day-to-day care. Unless the practitioners approve the theories they are required to use and have an understanding of their advantages and limitations, then they will be unable to illustrate the theories' worth to patients, colleagues, learners and other members of the multi-disciplinary team.

Practitioners should feel empowered by the theories they select, and they and their patients should have ownership of them. By using their power to impose a theory on practising nurses, managers and academics are being allowed to define expert nursing (Meave, 1994).

Philosophy as a guide for theory selection

In Chapter 4 the philosophy of scientific revolutions as propounded by Thomas Kuhn was discussed. To recap: Kuhn argued that science progresses through a series of revolutions where the old order of thinking is replaced by a new perspective. This is followed by a period of relative theoretical harmony which Kuhn referred to as 'normal science'. During this period one paradigm (Kuhn, 1970) or disciplinary matrix (Kuhn, 1977) rules supreme and practitioners, researchers, educators and managers work within this paradigm, adopting its lexicon and having faith in its ability to explain phenomena of concern to the discipline. At some stage a crisis occurs, when it becomes obvious that the ruling paradigm is incapable of dealing adequately with important issues. As a result, it comes under scrutiny and its supreme status is challenged by competing paradigms. The result of this revolution is the adoption of a new paradigm and a further period of normal science.

Kuhn (1970) asserts that the new paradigm does not build on the old one; science is not cumulative. Those interested in how the new paradigm is selected from among the competing paradigms may wonder how the choice is eventually made. Kuhn (1977) believes there are no universal rules for such a choice. Rather, the selection criteria vary from discipline to discipline and from time period to time period. Furthermore 'the [selection] criteria are always imprecise' (Kuhn, 1977: 321).

This imprecision can also apply to the way practising nurses select theories to guide their practice. Here too, there are only broad guidelines and no precise criteria. Very often the decision is a pragmatic one, where the issue for consideration is whether the theory is a realistic alternative to that which exists currently. For example, nurses working with terminally ill patients may realise that the medical model, with its emphasis on cure, is no longer appropriate. In their view, it does not deal with the very important psychosocial and spiritual concerns of the dying person, and a 'goodness of fit' crisis occurs. As a result, they begin examining other, more humanistic, nursing theories. This may be perceived as a Kuhnian revolution leading to a period of normal science where the new nursing theory guides practice, education and enquiry on the unit. If, two years later, a further crisis occurs as the chosen theory fails to answer new clinical questions or fails as a guide to new clinical situations, then other theories may be examined with the view to a further revolution. Here, the choice is based on practice rather than on a love of theoretical exploration, and the practical issues guiding the choice may be so diverse as to make it impossible to identify explicit selection criteria.

Other philosophies of science may exert influence on the selection of theories for practice. Cartesian rationalism, for instance, would indicate that the theorist developed his or her conceptualisations without having access to the clinical area. These so-called armchair theorists used reason to formulate their theoretical propositions. If practitioners were attracted to this method of theorising, then such theories may be the focus for choice. In contrast, empiricism means that the theory was developed inductively from experience within the patient care setting and the theory would be composed of concepts and propositions which represent what the theorist perceived through his senses. A theory developed in this way may have credibility with practising nurses and may therefore be a more appropriate choice for application in patient care. Historicism as an approach to theory development shows that the theorist has concentrated on the history, experiences, values and beliefs of those who underwent care and those who delivered care. Those nurses who value subjectivity and experience rather than objectivity and measurement would find these theories an attractive option.

Because of the power imbalance inherent in theory selection (see above) the critical science philosophy may usefully be employed as a means of selecting a suitable theory for practice. A nursing theory developed using this approach would be based upon the view that humans are typically dominated by social conditions that they can neither understand nor control and that enlightenment can free and empower them. This theory would be fervently against the medical model approach to nursing and could be attractive to nurses who perceive themselves as being disempowered by traditional approaches to care.

As a philosophy of science pragmatism may entice practitioners who wish to select a nursing theory for their practice. Essentially, pragmatism is concerned with the clarity of ideas and the value of these ideas when judged by their practical consequences. It calls for the clear and unambiguous use of words. It also argues that theory and knowledge are of little value unless they are useful in practice. To the pragmatist, if a theory cannot provide evidence of worthwhile outcomes then why select or use it?

Issues for consideration when selecting a suitable theory

The importance of theory to practice is becoming increasingly realised and a new awareness exists as to the necessity of making an appropriate choice. However, considering that there are approximately fifty grand nursing theories available, with little research as to which is the most effective, choosing between them is a daunting task and must be carried out with care.

Openshaw (1984) provides an excellent overview of how practising nurses make decisions. She examined several studies and theories on this subject and concluded that little is actually known about the complex processes involved in decision making. Several factors, including intelligence, expectations, memory and information overload affect an individual's decision-making ability. It is also possible that, when faced with different options, the decisions people make are influenced by how the options are presented. For instance, Tversky and Kahneman (1981) presented health care personnel with a decision task concerning two alternative immunisation programmes against a lethal disease. They found that wording the problem from a statement of lives saved to one of lives lost produced differing results. Therefore, decisions made regarding the selection of a nursing theory may be influenced by the language of different theories and how they are presented to practising nurses. This issue will be developed further when parsimony is addressed below.

Vinokuv (1971) formulated models of decision making based upon the work of Lewin (1951). Vinokuv believed that in making a decision between two or more courses of action it is rational to seek the maximum benefit to oneself. When faced with alternatives, the rational individual chooses the alternative with the most desirable outcomes. Therefore, it is possible that when nurses are selecting a nursing theory they will choose one that will suit their needs rather than those of their patients.

Borrowed or unique theory?

An important issue to consider when selecting a theory for nursing is whether we should borrow theory from other disciplines. Johnson (1968) defined 'borrowed theory' as that knowledge that is developed in the main by other disciplines and is drawn upon by nursing. In contrast, 'unique theory' is that knowledge which nurses derive from the observation of nursing phenomena and the asking of questions unlike those asked by other disciplines.

Kikuchi and Simmons (1992) maintain that questions concerning whether or not nursing knowledge is borrowed or unique have disappeared from the nursing literature. However, they discussed borrowing at length in their 1994 text, where they argued that if the central concerns of nursing are not identified then nursing problems will continue to be directed and studied through the lenses of other disciplines, or nurses will study that which is of central concern to other disciplines. The upshot of this, they assert, is that the unique knowledge required to improve nursing practice will not be developed.

Nurses who wish to select an appropriate theory for practice may ask themselves the following questions. If we select a borrowed theory will we be advancing nursing knowledge or the knowledge base of the other discipline? Alternatively, if we select a unique nursing theory will this place restrictions on our practice and will it cause communication problems with other disciplines?

Donaldson and Crowley (1978) admit that knowledge from other disciplines is very important for nurses' social understanding. But, in many instances, nurses do not bother to adapt borrowed theories. This often results in theory that is incomplete and poorly representative of any philosophy of nursing care. Slevin (1996) discussed 'theory adoption' and 'theory adaptation'. Theory adoption is where a theory is taken wholesale and used without it being altered to suit the new situation to which it is being applied. Nurses' use of classical conditioning theories from psychology is an example of this. Theory adaptation is where the theory is taken and moulded to suit the new situation.

Walker and Avant (1983) identified a process called theory derivation. It is composed of the five steps shown in Box 5.1 opposite.

This process leads to theory which differs from borrowed theory in that it involves an alteration of the content or structure of the existing theory, whereas borrowed theory is not modified.

Therefore, perhaps borrowed theories are only acceptable when it is not the theory that is important but the depth, blend, perspective

***Box 5.1* Walker and Avant's five steps for theory derivation**

1 Immerse oneself in the literature concerning the phenomenon/problem of interest in nursing and evaluate the suitability of existing theories to explain the phenomenon.
2 Analyse the literature from other disciplines to identify possible analogies.
3 Choose a parent theory from the other disciplines to transpose and reformulate in order to explain the phenomenon of interest in nursing.
4 Identify the content or structure from the parent theory that will be used in nursing.
5 Modify the concepts from the parent theory and restate the concepts in the form of propositions to derive theory for nursing.

and application of the theory. Borrowed knowledge can be refined, transformed and tested for its relevance to the goals and concerns of nursing. Folta (1971) states that nurses should select borrowed but relevant theories and order them in unique patterns in the light of professionally established hierarchies of relevance, appropriateness and social value. By doing this, borrowed knowledge, through transmutation, becomes nursing knowledge. According to McKenna (1993: 126), when this occurs borrowing from different disciplines is 'one of nursing's greatest strengths'.

None the less, it is worth being cautious: nurses should be careful to avoid the temptation of borrowing from other disciplines without first investigating what those theories have done for those disciplines. In addition, because borrowed theories may need to undergo intensive reworking to fit nursing's unique perspective, borrowing may not be as simple a process as it first appears – we could end up with an invalid and unreliable hybrid.

Another view is that we should not be worried about ownership, because theories belong to the scientific community at large not to one particular discipline. In 1968 Johnson asserted that discovery does not confer the right of ownership. The same year Rosemary Ellis (1968: 222) stated that 'theory, whether begged, borrowed, derived or originated by nurses, is significant if it can enlighten [nursing] practice'. Dickoff and James (1971: 501) concur with this perspective. They argue that it is the output for practice that is relevant, not some notion of originality or a contribution to a unique body of knowledge. They call for 'this foolish emphasis on idiosyncrasy in concept, method or definition' to be abandoned in favour of more relevant concerns of practice. Stevens-Barnum (1994) agrees, believing that knowledge is shared not borrowed, and that such shared knowledge has made an important contribution to modern nursing.

Perhaps we worry unnecessarily about borrowed knowledge. Fry (1992) states that nurses have consistently borrowed not only theories but methodologies from other disciplines. This is acceptable because very few professions can claim that their knowledge is not borrowed. Levine (1995) points out that there is not a nursing theorist who does not have a debt to other disciplines, even those who will not admit it. She states that turning psychological concepts into nursing concepts does not eliminate the debt.

This eagerness to 'go shopping' for borrowed theory is not a strategy supported by every nurse. Thirty years ago, Wald and Leonard (1964) argued that if practitioners continued to borrow theories from other disciplines, research problems based upon these theories would be phrased as questions that have little to do with nursing. More recently, Smith (1990) has supported this assumption. She warns that borrowing means returning. The borrower returns the fruits of the knowledge development to the discipline from which it was borrowed. For instance, using and testing sociological theories within nursing may do more for the knowledge base of sociology than for nursing. Smith called for the development of unique theories rather than trying to make borrowed theories fit.

Referring to mental health nursing, Phil Barker (1991) states that the continued influence of traditional viewpoints expressed through biological, psychodynamic and behavioural models (*sic*) are unhelpful. These models are more concerned with control than understanding. They emphasise repair work (Barker 1991: 38).

Earlier, Reed (1987) argued that while non-nursing theories provide valuable knowledge for practitioners, they may be incongruent with or limit nursing's perspective of significant care issues. Accordingly, she suggests that only unique nursing theories offer a means of clarifying nursing's conceptual base.

Adam (1992) also takes this stance, maintaining that nursing science can only advance if knowledge is built from a nursing frame of reference. She warns us that selecting non-nursing theories encourages nurses to identify with other disciplines, adding that for this reason the unification and advancement of theory development in nursing is unnecessarily limited. To a large extent this corresponds with the picture in allied health professions. Social workers, for instance, began with an adherence to the medical model only to supplant it with theories of their own as the discipline evolved. Freed too from the perceived shackles of the medical model, nursing leaders have communicated the need for the development of theory that is 'not just relevant but basic' to their practice (McFarlane 1986a: 72).

This call for a continuation in the development of unique nursing theories is still strong. Huch (1995) relates how a panel of well-known theorists strongly rejected Meleis's (1991) call for nurses to get involved in multidisciplinary theorising. They asserted that nurses should adhere to the goal of developing theory specifically for nursing practice and continue to build up their own knowledge base as other disciplines do. They predicted that it may not be long before other health care disciplines begin to borrow theories developed by nurses. There is some evidence to suggest that occupational therapists and physiotherapists are borrowing and reformulating nursing theories (e.g., self-care and activity-of-living theories) for their practices.

Level of practitioners' knowledge

Susan Gadow (1990) points out that nurses tend to consult outside experts when they should look to each other for judgement and guidance. But I wonder how realistic it is for us to expect the busy practitioner to be *au fait* with more than a few grand nursing theories. The level of knowledge about different theories will influence the appropriateness of the one chosen. For instance, Minshull *et al.*'s (1986) human needs theory may be a perfect fit for a particular clinical area, but if the staff are unaware of its existence it will not be considered as a suitable choice.

This knowledge deficit may be helped by bridging the theory–practice gap between what practitioners know and the theories nurse educators teach. If a theory being used on the wards is not the one favoured by the nurse educators who teach the students, the theory–practice gap can be perpetuated. But involving educators in the selection process may not necessarily be the answer, for there is yet another theory–practice gap: I refer to the gap between what theorists write and debate and what educators know and teach. Levine (1995) warns that if nurse educators are indifferent about nursing theory then students will sense this and leave theory behind when they become practitioners. So, perhaps practitioners are hindered in their choice of theory by two theory–practice gaps rather than one.

An eclectic approach to theory selection

Eclecticism means choosing what is best from different sources, systems or styles. This suggests a selector-preference scale rather than any particular standard based on external criteria (McGee, 1994). It is very attractive to indulge in eclecticism; the restrictions are minimal and the feelings of uncertainty are reduced because it is comfortable to use bits and pieces from what are available and familiar. With eclecticism, the influences of a selector's culture and context dictate in no small measure what is selected.

McGee (1994) defines eclecticism as the fortuitous use of a variety of components, concepts and elements from a range of theoretical constructs or models, to facilitate practice at a given point in time. This means that eclecticism encourages one theory of practice that changes with every practitioner in every situation and one that consists of elements, components and processes that have found favour with the clinician. While eclecticism could relieve the pressures on practitioners to conform to one theory of nursing or to learn several theories thoroughly, it could be argued that it brings nursing a step nearer to a unified theory sought after by so many colleagues (McGee, 1994).

This idea that different concepts can be chosen from several theories and applied in the clinical area as one theory is supported by some (Fawcett 1980), but regarded as totally untenable by others. Webb (1986a) argues that such a strategy would lead to the loss of coherence and rigour, the introduction of contradiction, and theoretical status being compromised. For example, if research results indicated that Roy's theory was a valid choice for intensive care nursing, this validity might be compromised if it was merged with Roger's theory and Neuman's theory. Practitioners could be left with an invalid, unreliable and unresearched hybrid theory. Furthermore, no construct validity can be argued for such a hybrid theory because the bits and pieces may not be compatible. Therefore, whether pieces of one grand theory can be amalgamated legitimately with another to guide practice is open to question (McGee, 1994).

Clare (1976: 64) recognises certain dangers with the eclectic approach. He believes that it is the soft option of 'a wishy-washy gutless mind that lacks decisiveness and clarity'. In this regard he was echoing the views of Eysenck (1971), who criticised those who subscribed to a 'mish-mash' of theories. In addition, if the mixed and matched ingredients of an eclectic theory are treated like a stew it could weaken curricula and practice. Dickoff and James (1982) warned against such a trial-and-error approach to theory selection.

However, there may be good reasons for adopting an eclectic stance. In Britain, Altschul (1980) recommends that, in the complex field of mental health, no one theory is always appropriate and nurses should use skills based on whatever approach they regard as helpful to a particular situation. Correspondingly, Reed (1987) argues that normally, when caring for a patient, nurses tend to use information from all the available theories.

In order to survive in a continually changing world, nursing should be open to modification and improvement. The use of one static theory would be proscriptive, narrow and counter to the philosophy of holistic care-giving. Furthermore, theories may be a product of their social context and some former thinking, becoming inappropriate over time. There may also come a point when an eclectic theory will fit a situation so well that it will no longer be an eclectic theory, rather it will be a new theory in its own right.

Ethical issues

Carper's (1978) 'ethical knowing' affects the choice of a theory. Selection is value-laden and nurses' choice of an appropriate theory will be influenced by their values and beliefs about the nature of people and health care. For example, if you value the idea that all ill people should be dependent and do as little for themselves as possible then you would not select a self-care theory. Further, when taking a decision to choose Orem's self-care theory, practitioners may also have to consider whether they should encourage all patients to be self-caring and whether they will put a boundary on how far self-care can go (e.g., would they allow a patient to get their own medicine out of the drug cupboard?). They must also consider whether encouraging self-care and family care will lead to fewer nurses being employed.

McKenna (1993: 124) believes that in order to influence nursing practice successfully, theories must focus on what is 'ideal', but be sufficiently credible and in touch with reality to make the 'ideal', or movement towards it, seem achievable. This exhortation seems to suggest that nurses should select an ideal theory on the grounds of whether or not it could eventually influence practice. However, Hardy (1986) questions the ethics of selecting an ideal theory that can promise more for patients than nurses can at present provide, and suggests that building up the patient's hopes by setting idealistic goals is morally indefensible.

In America, Jensen (1973) fooled many government officials with his theory that black children were less intelligent than their white counterparts. Similarly, a recent publication by Lynn (1996) puts forward the theory that male university students are more intelligent than female university students. This represents 'theories as ideologies', and the selection of such theories to frame policy or practice would have negative implications for hiring employees, for providing educational opportunities and on the self-esteem of many people. The dangers of rigid preference and application of any theory must be realised; the theory that the earth was flat and that the sun orbited the earth, for example, led to Galileo being victimised.

Social and political issues

Social and political implications also have a role to play in the selection of an appropriate theory (Rogers, 1986). The many theories that currently exist compete for advocates and supporters. Nurse teachers typically vote for their favourite one, which then serves as a guide for their curricula. Practitioners, too, vote or select one from several to guide their work. Schlotfeldt (1992) asks whether what is, in essence, a philosophical question concerning the nature of nursing should be answered by political pressures, by vote, by mandate.

It may not be possible to divorce theory selection from political issue, however. Webb (1986a) asserts that Orem's work is more suitable to the private health insurance sector because of its emphasis on the client's ability to undertake self-care as soon as possible. There is yet another element to this argument. If we commit ourselves to promoting adaptation, independence or self-care, we will be held accountable by society for this particular service. The philosopher Paul Feyerabend (1977) has argued that theory and truth cannot be divorced from the social and political context in which they exist. He asserts that the theory one chooses is a matter of social convenience or political expediency.

Currently, European governments are being encouraged to reduce the number of hours worked by junior doctors. There is much debate on whether the medical duties left undone as a result of this reduction should be taken up by nursing staff. Greenhalgh & Co. (1994), in a report commissioned by the UK government, stated that there are many technical procedures normally undertaken by junior doctors which could easily be carried out by nurses. This political initiative could encourage many nurses to revisit and reselect the medical model and to leave behind more patient-centred nursing theories.

The world is changing, and a theory which was useful yesterday may not be useful today or tomorrow. Contemporary nurses are working collaboratively in multidisciplinary teams – the choice of a unidisciplinary theory may be inappropriate. Nurses are also being faced with an increase in technology, so the choice of a theory that ignores technology may also be inappropriate.

Furthermore, nurses are increasingly focusing attention on families and community groups, so the choice of a theory that concentrates on providing care solely to individuals may be inappropriate.

Intuitive or scientific selection

Should the selection of a theory be based upon scientific enquiry or merely the 'gut reaction' of the nurse? In attempting to answer this question Mary Silva (1977) urged practitioners to value truths arrived at by intuition and introspection as highly as those arrived at by scientific experimentation. In contrast, Kikuchi and Simmons (cited in McGee, 1994) warn that if nursing theories are selected according to individual preferences rather than a standard, nursing's efforts to create a scientific knowledge base will remain fragmented. Supporting this, Aggleton and Chalmers (1986) stress that preferences must be made on logical scientific grounds. None the less, perhaps Silva's assertion is a valid one: after all, in most cases within nursing the theory exists before the research to test it is carried out.

The use of multiple theories

Although some authors maintain that most theories are applicable to any setting (Lister, 1987), the choice of just one theory for uniform application throughout an area of practice is seen as imprudent (McKenna, 1989). Should clients and practitioners have to put up with one theory that has a less desirable 'fit' for the sake of conformity? In such a case, most client-care information would be forced to fit into unsuitable theoretical categories, while for some there will simply be no category available. In addition, individual nurses have unique experiences, knowledge and skills. To constrain these within one theory would return nursing to the procedure book and medical model mentality of the past.

There exists, therefore, a body of opinion that strongly stresses the need to employ different theories to suit different client settings (Stevens-Barnum, 1994; McKenna, 1989). After all, most advanced practice professions have multiple theories that make up what may be referred to as their 'theoretical tool-kit'. Nurses, too, should have access to many theories, simply because there is no one theory that fits every clinical situation.

According to Koziel-McCain and Meave (1993) we must give up the struggle to select one theory which will provide us with certainty; rather, we must discover and embrace the richness of diversity. Echoing this, Levine (1995) states that such diversity is a major strength within nursing. However, to introduce a note of caution: it is one thing to say that diversity is necessary if we are to make progress; it is quite another to say that only diversity of thought is to be pursued and that all the different points of view are equally valid and must be respected as they stand (Kikuchi and Simmons, 1994).

McGee (1994: 64) defined theoretical pluralism as 'the acceptance and selective utilisation of the models and theories of nursing science to describe, explain, predict and or prescribe nursing process and outcome in terms the situation dictates'. But, while being a theoretically pluralist discipline is a proud boast, we must be aware that, without a clear and coherent philosophy of nursing, there is the danger of conceptual murkiness.

Furthermore, although the selection within one hospital of different theories for different client settings may be a desirable and recommended stratagem, it could lead to great problems with in-service training and documentation. It may compound communication problems: those who would be 'crossing the lines' between different areas, such as managers, tutors and paramedical staff, would require a high degree of theoretical sophistication. To the uninitiated, such a client-care system could resemble a conceptual Tower of Babel.

Length of client stay

Time is an important factor when choosing a theory. When one is working within a relatively short time frame, for example, in a casualty or an acute admission ward, FANCAP (the concise assessment framework: F = fluids, A = aeration, N = nutrition, C = communication, A = activity, P = pain) (Walsh, 1991) might be more suitable than a complex theory such as Roy's (1970) adaptation theory. Moreover, patients are spending less time in hospital and day surgery is increasing in frequency. This has implications for the theories that nurses select. Hospital nurses have less time to get to know the patient and so detailed interpersonal theories may not be appropriate. Community nurses are looking after more seriously ill patients than they have done in the past and therefore their theoretical focus is also changing.

Restrictiveness of theories

In discussing the application of theories, Smith (1986) concludes that each theory is limited by its own assumptions and therefore no one theory will be able to deal with all eventualities. Some nurses want assurance that a so-called 'right choice' of a theory would eliminate all their client-care problems. But it is possible that the inherent restrictions in individual theories may burden nurses with too narrow a perspective. For example, we cannot be criticised for failing to emphasise self-care if the theory we are using stresses the manipulation of stimuli to promote adaptation. Furthermore, as mentioned in Chapter 4, while we berate the medical model for reducing people to anatomical parts and physiological systems, we should remember that by selecting Roper, Logan and Tierney's (1990) or Roy's (1970) theories we are reducing patients to twelve activities of living or four adaptation modes respectively.

Making a wrong choice

Mistakenly choosing an inappropriate theory may also have undesirable consequences. Aggleton and Chalmers (1986) believe that the quality of care would be adversely affected, while McKenna (1994a) maintains that early closure on an unsuitable theory may stifle creativity. But, although an unsuitable choice is regrettable, nurses can always force a Kuhnian revolution and select another, more appropriate theory. To support this, Clark (1986) maintains that, if a theory does not fit comfortably, it should be discarded like an ill-fitting pair of shoes.

Staff attitudes

Loughlin (1988) claims that there exists at clinical level a distrust of theories. Hawkett (1989) argues that practitioners view theories with suspicion and describe them as 'woolly and impracticable'. Such negative attitudes are possible influencing factors on the 'unbiased' selection of theories for nursing practice.

McKenna (1992) found three main types of attitude towards nursing theories. First, he encountered fear and uncertainty. Practising nurses were concerned that these theories were fine for students in a classroom but that in the ward they were going to show qualified staff in a poor light. If we return to the metaphor of theories being like maps to guide our practice, novices require these maps because they are in unfamiliar terrain. However, as with the native of a town, experts do not need maps; they have internalised their own through their experience. In other words, by introducing the new theory, expert practitioners could be made to look like novices. The best strategy here is to assure these nurses of support and education and to allay their fears.

The second attitude McKenna came across was one of resentment and anger. Here, practitioners expressed distrust and were willing at every opportunity to sabotage the selection and use of the theory. The best strategy in such cases is to involve these nurses in the introduction of the theory. Finally, McKenna met nurses whose attitudes reflected interest and a desire to become involved in choosing and applying the theory. The best strategy in these instances was to encourage involvement in an atmosphere of realism and to promote a healthy scepticism that the theory might well not offer a remedy for all their clinical problems.

Multidisciplinary theories

Modern health care is a multidisciplinary endeavour and a team activity and therefore doctors, physiotherapists, etc. may also have a view on how the patients are being nursed. In such a culture, nurses are being seen increasingly as team players. In the not too distant future we may begin to value, select and use multidisciplinary theories on pain, rehabilitation and pre-operative care. Considering this, Smith (1994) believes that the uniqueness of nursing knowledge is no longer a relevant question for the 1990s. She maintains that human concerns will be investigated through a multidisciplinary lens, blurring, perhaps even dissolving, the once sacrosanct disciplinary boundaries. By focusing on distinguishing our beliefs, values and theories, nurses may cause false dichotomies that will not merely limit their perspective but will divide them. Smith (1994: 50) calls for a relational rather than a divisive approach in order to avoid the situation of nurses 'flourishing in a dissensus rather than consensus'.

Grand, mid-range or practice theories

Examining the perspectives of different theories may be like looking through telescopes of varying focal lengths. Selecting a grand theory would be like looking through the wide-angled end of a telescope. Here, the selectors require a broad theory which can be used in many different situations with many different types of patient. While the grand theory will not specify explicit interventions, it will give them a framework for viewing the world and an assessment template for practice. Selecting a mid-range or practice theory would be like focusing a telescope on a particular nearby scene, where more detail is observed but the surrounding landscape cannot be seen in its entirety. Here, a theory is required for a particular patient-care situation and in the case of a practice theory a guideline is presented for nursing action. Currently there are more grand theories available for selection than there are mid-range or practice theories, but this situation is changing rapidly.

Criteria for selecting an appropriate theory

Audrey Miller (1989) states that when selecting a nursing theory the relevance to practice is central. She suggests that the person who is choosing the theory should seek answers to the following questions:

● Does the theory have direct relevance for the way in which nursing is practised?
● Does the theory describe real or ideal care?

- Have its assumptions and propositions been tried and tested?
- Does it deal with the resources which are necessary for good care?
- Does it guide the use of the nursing process?
- Does it provide practising nurses with good direction for clinical actions?
- Are the concepts within the theory too abstract to be applied in practice?
- Is the language of the theory easy to understand?
- Does the theory coincide with the practising nurse's 'know how' knowledge?

Afaf Meleis (1991) identified six criteria which she believes can be used as a guide for selecting a suitable theory for a clinical area.

- *Personal*: individuals discuss their personal comfort with the theory, their intuitive feelings and the theory's congruency with their philosophical view of life.
- *Mentor*: there are nurses who select a particular theory because they were mentored by the theorist. These nurses speak of the personal influence, respect, personal contact and educational experience of such mentoring.
- *Theorist*: who theorists are, their reputation and standing in the field, their status and how well they are recognised were also important indicators for the selection of a theory.
- *Literature support*: some nurses identified the availability of extensive writings about the theory, as these had assured them of the significance of the theory and the standing it had within that specialty.
- *Socio-political congruency*: this is similar to the previous point. Nurses reported preferring a particular theory because it merged with the current social and political climate; as such, it did not require structural changes nor did it necessitate a lot of preparation and it was not imposed by management.
- *Utility*: the ease by which a theory was understood and applied prompted a group of nurses to select it over another more complicated theory.

Meleis (1991) realised that selecting a theory was a subjective as

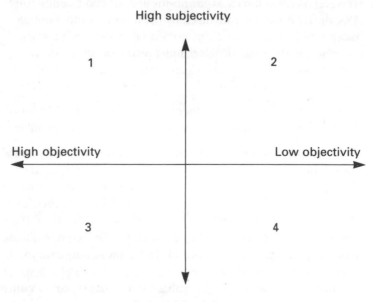

High subjectivity

1   2

High objectivity   Low objectivity

3   4

Low subjectivity

Figure 5.1   The subjectivity–objectivity selection continua

well as an objective process. In her opinion, the decision could fall
on two continua ranging from high to low objectivity and high to
low subjectivity (see Figure 5.1). Therefore, a choice made in quadrant 2 would be based on a high-subjective, low-objective decision,
while a choice in quadrant 3 would be based on a decision which
was low on subjectivity and high on objectivity. In the former case,
intuition plays a major role while, in the latter, rigid criteria are
used in the selection process. This latter approach may result in
the selection of an unpopular theory, especially if it is not congruent with the practitioner's perceptions of what nursing is really like.
    Meleis states that

    the subjectivity in theory selection is as important as the
    objectivity. We can select a theory based on well-defined cri-
    teria; therefore, the decision becomes highly objective.

However, if the theory's assumptions are not congruent with ours, or if we are not convinced by the theorist's experiential background, or if we are not comfortable with other work done by the theorist, the decision process becomes subjective.

(Meleis, 1991: 215)

More recently, after a comprehensive search of the literature, McKenna (1994a) found the following selection criteria popular.

- *Type of client*: when considering theories for practice, nurses should not be too concerned with which theory is popular in their country or region, or whether nurse educators or nurse managers are committed to a particular theory; rather, they should be concerned with which is best for the needs of their clients. The most appropriate choice of any theory must be based on the practitioner's knowledge of those they care for. If a grand theory is what is required, then it must be general enough to deal with the many diverse situations nurses come across when dealing with a homogeneous group of clients. Alternatively, if a practice theory is required, nurses must ask if the theory will provide specific guidelines for achieving clients' goals.
- *Health care setting*: this second criterion is related to the first but concentrates on contextual factors in the nursing situation. Glaser and Strauss (1967: 237) state that 'theory must fit the substantive area in which it is to be used'. In the introduction to this chapter, I likened theories to maps that guide practice. To take this analogy a step further, we may assume that we require a different map to suit the specific terrain in which we find ourselves. Also in the introduction I pointed out the implicit assumption in the literature that nursing practice will differ when different nursing theories are used. However, there is no substantial evidence to prove that this is true. The constraints of the context of care and the resources available influence how nurses practise nursing probably far more than any nursing theory alone. Therefore, staff in different clinical settings should select a theory depending on the fit of that theory to the culture and function of that setting.

- *Parsimony/simplicity*: as with Occam's razor (see Chapter 4) parsimony means selecting the simplest theory that will do the job. There are complex idealistic theories such as that formulated by Rogers (1970) and there are less complex but realistic theories such as that put forward by Henderson (1966). Why select the former if the latter will suit your needs and those of the clients just as well? A good theory is made up of just the correct number of concepts and propositions; it is elegant in its simplicity.

- *Understandability*: although this concept relates closely to parsimony, it merits separate consideration. Levine (1995: 12) criticises theorists who add to the 'considerable burden of imprecision in the language of nursing . . . new words that are unfamiliar and not easily related to nursing activities'. How can practitioners select a theory for practice if they need a theoretical dictionary to decipher its essential components? So, a theory must be easily understood if it is to 'cut any ice' with the hard-pressed practitioner. One cannot easily use a theory if one cannot understand it. Jackson (1986) wondered what use elaborate lines and circles were if practitioners were unable to use them to guide their practice.

   According to Miller (1989: 57), 'Some theories are abstract fantasies which are patently unrelated to everyday nursing practice and impossible to apply in the context of care in which practising nurses work.' In Australia, Speedy (1989) points out that, as long as nursing theories are too vague and abstract to be applied, they will be useless in their role of informing practice. Such theories only encourage separatism between theorist and practitioner.

   If the concepts used to build a theory are imperfectly understood by the theorist, then practitioners will have difficulty using them. What use are theories that ask practitioners to manipulate stimuli unless more guidance is given about how this manipulation should take place (Gould, 1989)? However, in case we become overcritical of theory complexity, we should take cognisance of the words of the Irish orator Edmund Burke (1729–97): 'A thing may look specious in theory, and yet be ruinous in practice – a thing may look evil in theory, yet in practice be excellent.'

- *Origins of the theory*: if a theory has its basis in the 'know how' of practice it may be more attractive to hard-pressed practitioners. In contrast, a theory that was formulated by academic 'armchair theorists', who based their work on reasoning alone, may not be a credible choice. Credibility may increase if a theory was generated and tested *in practice* by practitioners. Therefore, when selecting a theory nurses should explore its research and practice origins. If a theory is not reliable and valid, then the practice being guided by that theory may be adversely affected.
- *Paradigms as a basis for choice*: as discussed in previous chapters, every nursing theory has its roots in one or more of the following paradigms: systems, interactional, developmental and behavioural. These world views can help nurses make some preliminary decisions about the type of theory that is most appropriate for their work. Maloney (1984) supports this, maintaining that practitioners espousing an interactional approach to human nature are unlikely to select a systems theory to guide their care processes.

  The totality and simultaneity paradigms may also be used as a basis of choice (Parse, 1987). If practitioners perceive people as having biological, social, psychological and spiritual parts and as continually being confronted by environmental change to which they must adapt in order to maintain health, then theories from the totality 'stable' would be the proper focus for selection. In contrast, if practitioners believe people are meaningful individuals who are much more than just the sum of their parts and who are in continuous and mutual interaction with the environment and for whom health is a set of values, then the simultaneity 'stable' would be the focus for their selection exercise.
- *Personal values and beliefs as a basis for choice*: Sarter (1991) points out that nursing theories are laden with philosophical assumptions. Therefore, selecting a theory for practice may be influenced by the values and beliefs of the selector. McFarlane (1986a: 3) argues that 'most [practitioners] have a rough picture of practice which includes ideas about the nature and role of the client and the nurse, the environment . . . in which practice

takes place, and the major field of function, i.e., health care and the nature of action.'

McFarlane's statement is an attractive one, since we all have a personal conception in our minds regarding the central components of our craft. This conception is based upon our values and beliefs and is borne out of our education and experience over a number of years. These values and beliefs have been referred to as the practitioner's implicit nursing theory (Kristjanson, Tamblyn and Kuypers, 1987). Therefore, practitioners have a personal theory that they use to guide their practice. These personal beliefs and values incorporate assumptions concerning the four metaparadigm elements of nursing, health, person and environment (Fawcett 1995). Nurses can use this as a template for selecting suitable theories.

If asked, most nurses are able to reveal these private images; however, in the reality of the practice situation they are seldom articulated. Rather, they are mostly hidden in the practitioner's mind and rarely made explicit (Clarke, 1986). Bishop (1986) also fears that these 'personal guides to practice' may be incomplete, unproved, inconsistent and muddled.

The internationally recognised nursing theories are by no means value-free. They too were initially founded on the 'private images' (Fawcett, 1980), 'individual views' (Smith, 1986), 'mental pictures' (Adam, 1980) and 'rich insights' (Bohny, 1980) of their originators. Invariably they also tend to concentrate on nursing, health, person and the environment, and the relationships between these elements.

In education, Argyris and Schon (1974) distinguish between 'theory of action', the formal theory that practitioners have adopted, and 'theory in use', the informal theory which they actually use in practice. In nursing this is also common. Officially, practitioners may appear to be using Roy's (1970) or Orem's (1980) theories, but unofficially they are using their own theory. The official theory is confined to the documentation and the ward office while the unofficial theory is confined to the nurses' hearts and minds.

Selection strategies

Adam (1980: 82) outlines five possible ways to select a suitable theory for practice:

- A committee or group makes their choice from existing theories;
- Every concerned individual participates in a comparative study of several theories;
- An entire group develops its own specific theory;
- A group chooses an existing theory, but plans to develop its own from that basis;
- 'Bits and pieces' are taken from several theories to form an 'eclectic' theory.

She points out that although the first two methods are lengthy processes, in the end the change will be more lasting if every individual concerned has been part of the decision-making process.

Based on using the metaparadigm as a criterion for selection, Fawcett (1989) offers the following strategy. She maintains that a practitioner's own beliefs and values about the person, the environment, health and nursing will direct them to look for a theory congruent with these ideas. In other words, accepting that every nurse has a personal perception of the metaparadigm components, and that recognised theories also have this focus, a practitioner can choose a grand theory that best reflects their beliefs and values related to these elements (McKenna, 1994a). This is an essential prerequisite if the theory is to fit the reality of practice. Mansfield (1980), when considering the selection of a theory for psychiatric nursing, wrote that although it is advisable to practise what we preach, it is difficult, if not impossible, to practise what we could not preach from the heart.

Webb (1986a) asserts that if practitioners cannot accept how some concepts are treated within a particular theory, they should reject that theory and choose another whose concepts would be more compatible with their own. In this way, congruence will be reached between the nurse's clinical orientation (theory in use) and a recognised theory (theory in action). Then the final choice will indicate for practitioners what they have always believed about their work but could not articulate in as clear and distinct a manner as could the selected theory.

McKenna (1989) used this strategy to help nurses in mental health settings to select an appropriate nursing theory. He extracted the metaparadigm components from nineteen published nursing theories and formulated a theoretical matrix (see Appendix). Ninety-two respondents were asked to read each one carefully, making a first and second choice of those that they believed to be suitable for the nursing care of their patients. They were informed that they had to choose a theoretical statement in its entirety. Each respondent was given an opportunity (if they so desired) to change their mind and reselect. In the original theoretical matrix the theorists' names were missing. This was done to avoid the possible bias of the respondent knowing particular theorists or their work. Most of the respondents selected the human needs theory of Minshull, Ross and Turner (1986).

Johnson and Baumann (1992) wrote of how they used a 'process-oriented approach' as a strategy to select a nursing theory for psychiatric nursing in a Canadian hospital. At the outset of the project they realised that busy practitioners would be overwhelmed by the number of theories available. They also felt that staff were anxious and uncertain as to how to commence the selection process. They planned to get a 'goodness of fit' between what the practitioners saw as important for practice and what published theories promised.

Johnson and Baumann (1992) state that practising nurses have three options open to them:

- They could continue to use a non-articulated personal theory, recognising that the opportunity to refine theory, strengthen practice and enhance the visibility of the nursing profession may be lost.
- They could select from current nursing theories one that resonates with their beliefs and styles of practice, modifying it to meet the needs of their specialty.
- They could develop, articulate and use their own nursing theory.

Johnson and Baumann (1992) decided to opt for the second strategy. They identified the following three phases:

1   *Setting the stage*
     Creating a climate conducive to change;
     Clarifying advantages of using a theory in practice;
     Identifying potential barriers to successful introduction.

2   *Articulating practice requirements*
     Describing the nurses' own values;
     Categorising the attributes of clients;
     Identifying effective interventions.

3   *Selecting and testing*
     Establishing goodness of fit;
     Using the theory on a trial basis;
     Developing a more relevant theory.

In 'setting the stage', Johnson and Baumann realised that, if the organisation was not prepared (owing to lowered responses, competing interests or more pressing priorities), then the selection procedure should be postponed until a more conducive climate is available. There were other possible reasons for postponement: other disciplines could resent or actively oppose nurses selecting a theory, or experienced staff could have good clinical skills but be uncomfortable with conceptualisation. Alternatively, recently qualified staff might be comfortable with conceptualisations but lack the depth and intuitive 'know how' of experienced staff. Johnson and Baumann (1992) feel that pluralism in the selection process is very important. Depending on specialty, culture and perspective of staff, several theories may be the preferred option.

   In 'articulating practice requirements', Johnson and Baumann (1992) recommend that nurses make explicit their own beliefs about nursing, health, the person and the environment. Themes should emerge and 'the more clearly these themes are articulated and the way in which they influence practice elaborated, the easier it will be for nurses to identify nursing theories that reflect a similar or compatible orientation' (1992: 10). Also in this phase, the importance of identifying the attributes of the clients and the clinical interventions used is highlighted.

   In the third phase, 'selecting and testing', a review of the literature is undertaken to identify a shortlist of nursing theories that appear to resonate best with the issues identified in the second phase. In this way, a 'goodness of fit' is achieved. Johnson and Baumann (1992) also suggest that because of the multidisciplinary nature of modern health care the selected theory should allow for a high degree of compatibility with the non-nursing theories being used in that setting. Finally, they realise that the selected theory may lack certain critical ingredients necessary to meet particular practice requirements and therefore should be adapted.

McGee (1994) recommends the following 'index of utility' as an appropriate strategy for selecting theories (see Figure 5.2). McGee believes that such selection criteria will avoid what Chinn and Kramer (1991: 15) call 'choices gone wild'.

Goodridge and Hack (1996) used a selection strategy based upon a quality improvement project in a 320-bed facility in Winnipeg, Manitoba. A central tenet of the 'continuous quality improvement' movement is the focus on organisational cultural change. They argue that the selected theory must be congruent with the organisational ethos. They also recognise that the allegiance to the theory would be short-lived unless the staff were able to implement it in a meaningful way in their daily practice. If not, they reasoned, the theory would exist on paper only. Therefore, in order to ensure adoption and integration into practice, the theory selection process had to be undertaken in a systematic and considered manner. A core belief of the project was that attempting to introduce a nursing theory which was at odds with the values and beliefs of the staff would be futile (Goodridge and Hack, 1996: 42).

Their selection strategy involved gaining a rich understanding of the professional culture of the nursing staff so that a strategic fit could be achieved with a relevant theory. Using the Nursing Unit Cultural Assessment Tool (NUCAT-2) they obtained a view of the cultural norms of the organisation and the staff therein. This was followed by the use of four focus groups which explored the meaning of the metaparadigm components – nursing, health, the person and environment. The end result was that they were able to reject many theories which were at odds with the staff and the organisation's cultural norms and how the staff viewed the metaparadigm. The study is ongoing.

```
A   Social value
Benefit to society:              high          medium        low
Explicitness of value
   assignment:                   precise       adequate      imprecise
Ethical decision guidance:       excellent     fair          poor
Conflict management
   guidance:                     excellent     fair          poor


B   Compatibility
With community culture:          high          moderate      low
With the health care system:     high          moderate      low
Between client and nurse:        high          moderate      low


C   Completeness
Guidance in situations of:       morbidity,    crisis, risk,  normalcy
        Pragmatic adequacy:      high          moderate      low
        Logical adequacy:        high          moderate      low
        Empirical adequacy:      high          moderate      low
        Predictability:          high          moderate      low


D   Skill requirements
Skill range:                     Psychomotor, interpersonal,  cognitive


E   Feasibility
Requirements for
        1   Resources
                Human:                by type and level
                Material:             by type
                Space:
                Time:
                Logistical needs:     by availability and accessibility

        2   Potential/actual evidence of:
                Effectiveness:        high      moderate      low
                Efficiency:           high      moderate      low
                Adequacy:             high      moderate      low
                Appropriateness:      high      moderate      low
```

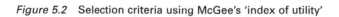

Figure 5.2   Selection criteria using McGee's 'index of utility'

Who should be involved in the selection process?

The literature is unclear about this, and merely suggests that practitioners be involved (Aggleton and Chalmers, 1986). Ellis (1969)
maintains that it is the professional practitioner who is able to criticise the theory and determine its value for directing actions to
achieve defined outcomes. In this 'she is not only a user of theory
but a modifier . . . and chooser of theory' (1969: 1435).

However, Pearson (1986) recommends that the clinical manager
of each unit should decide upon the most relevant theory. This
may indeed be a valid nomination considering that Kitson (1984)
identified the ward sister as possessing the most knowledge and
influence regarding clinical work orientation and practical expertise.

I was unable to find literature where the client was involved in the
selection of a nursing theory for practice. This is strange considering
the emphasis on the client as a partner in care. Since most theories
are normally formulated from the perspective of nurses not patients,
Hardy (1986) asks that the patient be actively involved in deciding
on an appropriate theory. Gould (1989) agrees, arguing that when
selecting a theory the beliefs and values of the most important person concerned, the recipient of care, cannot be ignored. None the
less, perhaps the following question merits consideration. If nursing
theories are viewed as confusing by many staff, would clients not
find them equally, if not more, confusing? If the answer is yes, then
one can see why there has been little evidence of partnership
between practitioners and clients in the selection of a theory.

To conclude, theories are like maps, and you will need a different
one depending on the territory in which you are working. The days
when managers and tutors chose theories for practice should now
be over. Clients should work alongside practitioners in the selection
process. If this occurs, the selected theory will be a realistic reflection of what those in practice and those in receipt of practice see as
important for patient care.

Summary

Because the choice of theory will affect how clients are assessed and
how care is planned and delivered, selection should not be a process

which staff undertake lightly. This chapter has identified several issues that must be taken into consideration when an appropriate theory is to be chosen. It has outlined a range of selection criteria and strategies which practitioners should find useful. The issues of who should make the choice and how this should be done are also addressed. In essence, there are many selection approaches available and nurses should not enter into the process without careful deliberation.

Chapter 6
Applying theories in practice

This chapter will concentrate on the application of theories to nursing practice. It will deal with the importance of applying theories in clinical settings and the effects this can have on quality of care. Barriers to using theory in practice will be explored, as will the roles that practitioners, managers, theorists and educators can play in encouraging the development and use of theory-based practice. The use of 'planned change' strategies will also be discussed.

It is a truism that theories are not being used in a systematic way to guide the delivery of client care. This is unfortunate, considering that theory does have important implications for the quality of patient care in that it aims to increase the sum of our knowledge so that the care of clients, their families and the public in general can be improved.

Lerheim (1991) used the metaphor of a coin, with one side being knowledge with its abstract concepts and theories and the other side being practice. She stresses that, like the coin, theory and practice are a unity and must be seen as a whole. However, considering that most of the grand theories used in nursing did not emanate directly from practice, one wonders if Lerheim is arguing for what should be the case rather than what is the case.

The relationship between theory and practice is reciprocal:

● Theory can grow and develop from practice;
● Theory can return to practice to be tested;
● Theory can act as a framework to guide patient care.

Many writers also acknowledge that the link between theories and practice is necessary for nursing's claim to be the provider of professional care. For instance, Chalmers (1989) argues that, without a strong orientation towards the work of theorists and the work of practitioners, the basic requirements for a profession are missing.

Botha (1989) supports this argument and goes further by stating that only if we are able to prove that this link exists will we be 'legitimate contenders' for professional status. However, based upon George Bernard Shaw's statement that 'professions are conspiracies against the laity', we could question whether professionalisation is in fact a desirable goal, considering that it may distance nurses from patients.

Interestingly, Smoyak (1988) challenges the necessity of a pragmatic link between theory and practice. She points out that some theories are not intended to be clinically relevant. She refers to Martha Rogers' theory (1970), suggesting that it is not meant for application in practice and that it never was. She quotes Rogers herself as saying that her theory is a stimulus for thinking and that it may even be dangerous to apply it directly to practice!

There is something attractive about this view. Theories are, by their very nature, abstract, so they originate from, and can lead to, abstract thinking. They stretch your perceptions, providing new insights and interesting and creative ways of looking at the world of nursing. That is part of their value. Since many are at the forefront of new knowledge development, they are extending the discipline's frontiers. Therefore, by definition, they cannot coincide with what is now being practised – to do so would limit their vision and restrict nursing within a time warp. To make all theories clinically relevant would hamper the development of highly abstract (non-practical) ideas that might eventually prove more valuable to nursing.

Alternatively, there is also attraction in the opposing position. Regardless of whether nurses work as researchers, educators, theorists, administrators or practitioners, it must be realised that they are in a practice profession with the client at the receiving end of that practice. Accepting this, theories should have a direct bearing on client care. If they do not, their value is open to question. To quote Perkins (1965: 421), 'if you know theory and not practice then you do not know the whole theory'.

Perhaps the true answer comes somewhere in between these two positions. Peter Draper (1991) would argue that there are two types of theory, the 'realistic', which coincide with the views of practitioners and current practice, and the 'idealistic', which may appear alien to contemporary practitioners. Pluralists may find solace in this second viewpoint. However, Draper states that an overemphasis on the importance of the latter group has hindered nurses' understanding of the real world of practice.

The theory–practice interface

There has been much written about the theory–practice gap (Nolan, 1989; Merchant, 1991). Here, theory may not necessarily mean the work of nurse theorists; rather, it can mean any types of 'know that' knowledge. Hunink (1995) outlined the following interpretations of theory:

1 Knowledge from books, instructions and guidelines for the practical situation;
2 As the opposite of 'practice' ('in theory' meaning – not in practice);
3. As a possible explanation, guess, assumption or hypothesis;
4 As a way of looking at something, a vision;
5 Scientific meanings, e.g.:
   ● a theory as a law, a universal rule (e.g., the law of gravity)
   ● as an explanation of a number of related facts
   ● as empirically tested knowledge or knowledge to be tested.

People who refer to the 'theory–practice gap' invariably mean the dichotomies that exist between what students are taught in classrooms and what they experience in clinical practice (items 1, 2 and 5 in Hunink's list). This may lead to 'cognitive dissonance', which is unsettling for individuals. For instance, without citing evidence, Clinton (1981) suggests that if students wrote down in an examination what they practised in reality, they would fail!

In Chapter 4, this theory–practice gap was conceived as a two-tier structure. On the first tier there is the gap between the up-to-date work of theorists and the theoretical knowledge that educators possess and teach, and on the second tier there is the gap between the theoretical knowledge that educators possess and teach and the theory that staff (including students) use in practice. There may even be a third gap, represented by the theory that staff use in the clinical area and the implicit theories that patients and the public in general have about nursing, health and social care.

In many cases it is apparent to qualified practitioners that their methods of planning and delivering care bear little resemblance to what the theories in journal articles or textbooks suggest. Miller (1985) was amazed by how academically distant Diploma in Nursing care plans were from normal practice. This is still the case in many nursing colleges. Students are encouraged to write comprehensive care plans using, for example, Roy's (1970) adaptation theory. This means writing many pages of text relating to the four adaptation modes, identifying focal, contextual and residual stimuli and the decisions about cognator or regulator influences. Care plans like this have limited uses in the real world of a busy surgical or medical ward, yet this is how students learn how to assess and plan care.

Perhaps, instead of bringing 'know that' knowledge and 'know how' practice closer together, theories may be doing the opposite. Biley (1991), for instance, stresses that nursing is still entrenched in traditional methods of caring and that the introduction of theories creates confusion and hostility, hence perpetuating the 'gap'. Furthermore, theories invariably come from an academic background and, as Jones (1990) states, most theorists have been away from practice and the reality of care for many years. Moreover, since most theories are not being formulated by or with practitioners or patients, this encourages the theory–practice gap to remain.

In America, Meleis (1991) felt that theorists were developing theories in isolation, researchers pursued questions of interest only to educators and administrators, while practitioners pursued their practices oblivious to what the other two groups were doing. Although Meleis writes in the past tense, there is little evidence to suggest that the situation has changed. But Rafferty, Allcock and Lathlean (1996) appear to suggest that we are unnecessarily perturbed by the 'gap'. They state that the theory–practice gap can never be sealed entirely; theories and practice are by their nature always in dynamic tension and this tension is essential for change in clinical practice (1996: 685). Therefore, the presence of a theory–practice gap may be a necessary stimulus for innovation in any discipline.

Whether or not we support this position may not be important. The theory–practice gap exists, has always existed and will continue to exist. While we accept this situation, every nurse's goal should be to spend a large part of their career trying to reduce it a little. We may be helped in this pursuit by considering the reasons for its existence. In 1981 Hunt gave five reasons why practising nurses do not use research. From the results of his study, McKenna (1994a) believes that these reasons can equally apply to the use of nursing theories in practice.

1 They do not know about them;
2 They do not understand them;
3 They do not believe them;
4 They do not know how to apply them;
5 They are not allowed to use them.

Theories applied in practice

The previous section described the reasons why theories are not applied in practice. Melia (1990) argues that the lack of application is a good thing, while Salvage (1990) stresses that clinical staff should not be made to feel guilty if their practice is not based on an explicit theory nor, she states, should it be assumed that all progressive practitioners are using one.

In the UK, research has shown that the theories most commonly used in practice are those of Roper, Logan and Tierney, Henderson, Orem and Roy (Mason and Chanley, 1990; McKenna, 1994a). These theories focus on the 'what' of practice rather than the 'how' or 'why' of practice. They are also firmly ensconced in the limiting totality paradigm (see Chapter 4).

Theories invented in an academic setting need considerable adjustment when applied to the vagaries of particular clinical situations. If this is not done and the theory is applied in a rigid fashion, the result may be confusion and apathy. However, we should be wary of making widespread alterations to a theory in case its original theoretical meaning is lost. As with selecting theories (see Chapter 5), taking an eclectic approach to theory application fails to recognise that concepts arise within the context of particular theories, and their meaning may be compromised if taken out of context and placed within a different theory.

As well as identifying the increase in paperwork as a problem, Pearson (1986) maintains that real practitioners caring for real clients are busy, tired, and therefore unable to engage in elaborate conceptual exercises throughout the working day. The perceived inflexibility and esoteric nature of some theories do not help the situation.

The question of whether we need one or many theories is equally relevant to theory application in practice. Most professions use several theories that show diverse views of the phenomena concerning their practice. For example, teachers use many theories of education; psychologists have many competing theories of behaviour; and sociologists extol numerous theories of the family. Similarly, the pluralism of theories within nursing is indicative of the current state of theorising in the discipline. In the first edition of their book Riehl and Roy (1974) advocated a single theory of nursing because such a theoretical approach would unify and lend stability to the profession. But Chapman (1990) claims that, since practice is becoming increasingly diversified and specialised, no single theory would be adequate to cover all care situations.

In the clinical area there are benefits and problems with using only one theory. For instance, Kristjanson, Tamblyn and Kuypers (1987) argue that the use of only one theory forces the practitioner to attend only to those things that the theory covers. In contrast, the application of more than one theory can lead to practical problems. As alluded to in Chapter 5, staff who move from ward to ward, such as bank staff, agency staff, tutorial staff, managers and students, would require a high level of theoretical sophistication to cope with the use of several theories in different care settings. Similarly, clients (and their families) who are transferred from hospital to community as their health state changes could be confused if their care was structured around more than one theory. There is also the problem of expense. If practitioners are required to use several theories, they need intensive in-service education to ensure competence in their application. Furthermore, different theories require different documentation for their application and this would lead to extra cost, as well as confusion.

For these reasons, it is felt that nursing as a discipline requires multiple grand theories while nursing within a discrete clinical area may find one grand theory sufficient, especially if it is selected and applied appropriately. Chalmers (1988: 16) maintains that one theory can be used in a particular unit for most of the people cared for there: she believes that 'individuality can be taken too far'.

Theories and the nursing process

Over the last two decades nurse practitioners in the United Kingdom have been taught and are being encouraged to use the nursing process. The 'process', as it is sometimes called, has at least four designated stages: assessment, planning, implementation and evaluation. As the logical steps in problem solving, all health care professionals use this four-stage process to identify client problems, plan solutions, implement the plan and evaluate whether the interventions have been successful. This begs the question: what makes the 'process' a nursing process rather than an occupational therapy process or a medical process? The answer is that it depends on the theory that is being used to structure and guide it. When car mechanics use the four-stage problem-solving approach within a mechanical theory they are using a mechanical process. Similarly, when nurse practitioners use the four stages within a nursing theory they are using the nursing process.

In the UK most nurses were introduced to the 'process' before they were aware of the existence of grand theories. This may account for the many problems encountered by clinical staff in the past when they attempted to apply the 'process'. Without a theory to underpin it, practising nurses did not know the who, when, why or what of assessing, planning, implementing and evaluating. It is noteworthy that the application problems have not disappeared now that nurses have got both theories and 'the process'.

Aggleton and Chalmers (1986) believe that using the nursing process without a theory is 'practising in the dark'. Continuing with the mechanical metaphor, if we take the engine and the bodywork of a car, the bodywork is of little use without the engine to drive it and the engine is also useless without the bodywork to house it. The nursing process is the engine that makes theories work in practice and the theories are the bodywork within which the nursing process functions.

Normally, theories of nursing are used as templates for client assessment. But Luker (1988) found that after the assessment the theory is forgotten and practitioners tend to rely on their pre-existing repertoire of interventions. This practice is unfortunate considering that the pre-existing interventions may be ritualistic and that most theories do offer broad guidelines for action. For example, Roper, Logan and Tierney (1983) suggest that practitioners should seek to prevent, solve, alleviate or teach the client to cope with problems with the activities of living. Orem's self-care theory (1980) suggests that practitioners use three different 'nursing systems' in order to support, create a better environment, or teach and encourage self-care. Therefore, we should not blame the theories for becoming redundant after the written assessment is complete; this trend is not their fault. The problems lie with the way that staff are applying theories to client care.

The effects of theories on quality of care

In the new health service of the late twentieth and early twenty-first centuries, health care professionals will have to show that they make a difference to the health care of the nation. They must focus on being effective as well as efficient. These are two of the hall-marks of providing a high-quality service. After undertaking a comprehensive trawl of the literature McKenna (1995) identified three major assumptions:

1   Nursing theories lead to better quality of care;
2   Nursing theories have an uncertain effect on quality of care;
3   Nursing theories lower the quality of care.

Nursing theories lead to better quality of care

Within the literature there are many writers who offer the unsubstantiated opinion that using theories would help to improve the quality of care. Fawcett (1989), for example, believes that the use of theories will foster a higher quality of practice than is evident when no explicit theory is used to guide activities. Similarly, McKenna (1995) found that most respondents were of the opinion that the most positive aspect of theories was their ability to improve the quality of care. Hawkett (1989) and Melia (1990) also thought that this would be the case.

A common argument put forward to support these opinions appears to be that theories provide practitioners with a knowledge base from which to give care (Chalmers, 1989). Other, more specific, reasons have been put forward: Meleis (1991) argues that a theory should improve quality because it clearly defines boundaries and goals, provides a guide to assessment, articulates actions, provides continuity and congruency in care, and allows for more accurate prediction of the range of client responses. Kershaw (1990) agrees, acknowledging that when practitioners use a theory there is little danger of them omitting vital aspects of intervention.

Theories are also said to improve the quality of care through leading to improved use of skills (Jones, 1990), through narrowing the theory–practice gap (Kershaw, 1986) and through leading to the setting of standards (Farmer, 1986). In addition, it is suggested that theories reflect individual differences in care (Chalmers, 1989), predict desired outcomes (Engstrom, 1984) and provide 'beginning criteria' for the evaluation of intervention outcomes (Fawcett, 1989).

Theories have an uncertain effect on quality of care

Some authors acknowledge that theories have an impact on quality of care but they do not state whether the impact is positive or negative. For instance, Webb (1986a) asked whether theories could influence the quality of care. In 1990 there were still many writers who could not or would not answer this question. They would rather reserve judgement on whether the effect of theories on quality was favourable or unfavourable. For instance, Walsh (1990) agrees that theories *should* improve care, but he is not sure if they do. Cash (1990) merely presumes that the attempts to implement theories have 'complex results' in terms of the quality of care delivered.

Theories lower the quality of care

It is interesting that this viewpoint is not encountered very often in the literature. Green (1985) acknowledges the possibility that theories do not improve the quality of care. She makes the proviso that it depends on the theory used. An example of Henderson's theory being applied in learning disability nursing is offered. Since this theory has a physiological basis and people with learning disability are not ill, she believes it would improve the quality of care but only in a limited way. Similarly, an esoteric theory like that of Rogers (1980) may cause such conceptual upheaval and confusion among practitioners that the quality of care could actually deteriorate. Furthermore, practitioners may spend so much time embroiled in the paperwork emanating from the use of a theory that actual care does not take place!

A grand theory may be viewed as a ladder by means of which we can climb from our immediate limited view of nursing to a position where we have a more panoramic vantage-point. Once we have reached this position, the ladder can be dropped or discarded. Gordon (1984) noticed that novices and beginners felt secure with theories to guide their practice. To some extent, the theories represented the solid rungs of the ladder that kept the student on the right route. However, expert nurses who have already reached the vantage-point no longer require the theory as a template for practice; like the ladder, it can be discarded. But later, if these expert nurses are asked to structure their care using a new theory, their practice skills will, initially at least, be slowed down to that of the novice. This may have detrimental effects on the smooth processes of care-giving and, ultimately, care quality.

Gould (1989) warns against applying a theory too rigidly. She wonders if staff can really give high quality of care when they are stuck with a theory that gives them no scope for innovation in practice. Collister (1988) also highlights the effects on care of applying theories like 'theoretical strait-jackets'. He points out that a theory is not a substitute for good care and that poor practice will not improve merely by using a theory.

Having considered all three assumptions, it would appear that those authors who are uncertain as to the effects of theories on quality of care may be correct in being non-committal. This is because, to date, there appears to be very little empirical evidence to confirm or deny that theories have a positive effect on care quality. This has been recognised after extensive research by Luker (1987), Chalmers (1988), Miller (1989) and McKenna (1995). There is of course a rapidly burgeoning body of research being undertaken into the effects of nursing theories. However, these tend to be small, poorly funded studies, and their non-cumulative nature is worrying.

Researching the effects of theories in practice

In 1990, British nurses like Girot, Burnard and Melia called for the major components within theories to be researched to see if they were more than the mere speculation of 'armchair theorists'. Earlier, Webb (1984: 22) had stated that these frameworks amount to no more than a collection of unverified assumptions which reflect the personal philosophies or value systems of their authors.

Whitehead (1933) stated that any science goes through three stages:

1　The stage of romance – ideas are explored and discussed in a fairly cavalier fashion.
2　The stage of precision – ideas are tested rigorously.
3　The stage of generalisation – general statements about the discipline can be made because of preceding research.

In examining the evolution of theories within these stages, Burnard (1990) maintains that nursing is 'stuck' at the stage of romance. None the less, Holden (1990) argues that, while it may not be possible to test scientifically the underlying assumptions and propositions of grand theories, it is possible to scrutinise certain aspects of care affected by their introduction. This call legitimised the carrying out of research to see if these conceptualisations had any effect on clients and their care.

Although grand theories are being used almost routinely by many nurses, there is, as alluded to above, very little research evidence available on the effects they have on client care.

Acknowledging this, Chinn and Jacobs (1987) in the US and Walsh (1990) in the UK recommend that research be carried out to determine the results of applying a theory in various care settings. In her British book about a 'research-based approach' to theories, Fraser (1996) notes that there is a plethora of articles and books on the application of theories and the positive effects that result from their use but few of these could be classified as research.

Webb (1986a) believes that until well-planned evaluative research is carried out it will be impossible to say whether it is the individual skill, knowledge and sensitivity of a certain nurse or the use of a particular theory which leads to quality of care. Until such research is available, we must rely on our own and others' subjective and impressionistic assessments of the benefits of using nursing theories (1986a: 174).

Similarly, Smith (1987) predicted that years from now nurse educators may turn everything on its head and state that nursing theories are a load of rubbish! However, to do so may prove extremely difficult if no written record has been maintained with the explicit purpose of evaluating progress (1987: 109). Here, you may legitimately question Smith's logic, as he felt the decision as to the value of nursing theories should be left to nurse educators!

Kershaw and Salvage (1986) called for an examination of the effects of theories on quality of client care, while Denyes *et al.* (1989) were more specific, suggesting measuring their effects on participants' satisfaction. Some researchers rose to this challenge. For example, in a small study at Guy's Hospital, London, Brewster, Cook and Woodward (1991) used Roper's theory as a basis for audit. They used the 'activities of living' elements from the theory to write twenty standards for a paediatric intensive care ward. Although strengthening the relationship between the two, this initiative does not establish a causal relationship between good practice and theories.

In midwifery there are few empirical studies relating to the effects of using theories in practice. In the UK, Midgley (1988) undertook a survey to note what nursing theories were being used in midwifery, rather than what effect these had. According to Midgley's research, Orem's (1980) theory was the most commonly used conceptualisation within midwifery. A recently published British text on theories in midwifery also failed to identify research into their effectiveness (Bryar, 1995).

Keyzer (1985), a British nurse tutor, used an action research approach to 'adopt' a nursing theory in practice and education. Keyzer used the 'observer as participant' role in four hospitals: one long-stay geriatric; one psychiatric rehabilitation; one community hospital; and one psycho-geriatric assessment unit. Findings suggested that, in the absence of a redistribution of power and control from managers, educators and doctors to practitioners and clients, the change to a theory-based practice would be difficult. Keyzer also stresses the importance of education programmes to support the change. Therefore, in order for the implementation of a theory to be successfully applied to practice, the relationships between nurse, client, relatives and managers would have to change (Keyzer, 1985).

In the US, Gordon (1984) employed anthropological methods of observations and interviews on two general surgical units to see if 'formal nursing theories' affected the way staff progressed from novice to expert. As outlined above, she found that such theories could be useful for new staff and students but that experienced staff may find them too constraining and reductionist. In Canada, the effects of the McGill University theory of nursing have been appraised in clinical practice. Studying the experiences of graduates using the theory, Gottlieb and Rowat (1987) state that it has achieved the following client outcomes: increased rates of satisfaction; decreased stress levels; increased problem solving; and increased involvement in health learning. It must be pointed out that the methodology used is not made explicit in Gottlieb and Rowat's paper.

Hoch (née Schmidt) (1987), in one of the few studies to use a quasi-experimental design, examined forty-eight retired individuals in Pittsburgh to see what effects the application of Roy's and Neuman's theories would have on their rates of depression and life satisfaction. Findings were highly significant, indicating that care based on the two theories resulted in lower depression scores and higher life satisfaction scores than did care based on no theory. Hoch does accept that the personal characteristics of the nurses may have influenced the results, and calls for the study to be replicated. One of her study's recommendations stresses that more research that tests the application of nursing theories to practice should be carried out (1987: 70).

Mason and Chanley (1990) found that 80 per cent of nurses in 'special hospitals' within the United Kingdom believed that nursing theories were ineffective; 5 per cent did not know; and 15 per cent said they were effective. None of the latter group could substantiate their positive view. Salanders and Dietz-Omar (1991) evaluated US nurses' perception of the utility of nursing theories after a two-year course. Findings indicated that the subjects believed that their decision-making skills concerning the planning and delivery of care had improved.

In a descriptive study, Lerheim (1991) surveyed twenty-eight experienced 'nurse leaders' in four Norwegian hospitals. Her goal was to see if the nursing service used 'nursing science' to develop and improve practice. She found that the impact of nursing theories was clearly expressed in a new independent attitude by practitioners. Lerheim concluded that theories are being used directly and indirectly to make a difference to practice. However, this was a small study and the findings may not be generalisable outside Norway.

It was pointed out previously that most of the literature on the application of nursing theories is composed of anecdotal care studies as opposed to rigorous research. While accepting the validity of this, there may be some benefits in practitioners writing about their experiences in applying theories. Roper, Logan and Tierney (1990) maintain that feedback from practitioners using their theory did provide the authors with a source of new ideas and highlight some of the application difficulties. Other theorists also found the subjective feedback from practitioners helpful (Roy, 1980; Orem, 1995).

McKenna (1995) undertook an action research approach to implement a nursing theory in a long-stay psychiatric area. The theory concerned was the human needs theory of Minshull, Ross and Turner (1986) previously selected by a population of ward managers (n = 95). Within a broader quasi-experimental design, specific quality of care indicators were appraised before and after the implementation of the theory. These dependent variables were also monitored on a control ward and data were collected on both wards at one pre-test and two post-test points. Planned change was used as a guiding framework for the implementation of the theory.

Results indicated that on the experimental ward there were statistically significant improvements in 'psychiatric monitor', clients' and staff's perception of ward atmosphere, client satisfaction, staff's views about nursing theories and client dependency levels. No significant changes were noted in practitioner satisfaction levels nor practitioners' perception of clients' behaviour. These findings suggest that, when implemented through an action research approach, where practitioners were involved as partners in the change process, a nursing theory has positive influences on the quality of client care.

But will such findings make any difference to future practice? Previously, Storch (1986) wrote that sceptics might find theory somewhat more palatable if they could be convinced that its application to practice can make a significant difference to the quality of client care. Green (1985) suggested that studies giving evidence of changes in the quality of care due to the implementation of a particular theory would make more interesting reading but, at that stage, she doubted if there were many such studies. It is also reasonable to suggest that nurses are no different from anyone else and that research evidence is not a good enough reason in many instances for changing established behaviour.

I am not calling for a moratorium on research into the effects of theory. In fact, considering the plethora of theories available, it is essential that studies continue to be carried out. However, as with all research, such investigations cost money. In the UK in the mid-1990s, not only is such funding difficult to obtain but also there are no easily identifiable sources for financing studies into the development, application or testing of nursing theory. It is also possible that in a more competitive and multidisciplinary-focused health service, funding for such projects may become even more difficult to obtain.

Roles and theory application

The role of practitioners in theory application

Unfortunately, practising nurses have some difficulty in justifying their actions by referring to a nursing theory. Though carried out in good faith, too often our interventions are steeped in tradition and passed down from one generation of nurses to another – often without theoretical substance. Jones (1990) suggests that the reason for this stems from practitioners seeing themselves as 'doers' and seeing theorists as 'thinkers'.

Since many nursing theories deal with what ought to be and not with what is, a dilemma is posed for practitioners who are more concerned with the 'is' of care and would feel more comfortable with a realistic theory that reflects the actuality of their practice. Therefore, nurses should seek compatibility between the formal theory and the practitioner's informal theory (McKenna, 1989). When such compatibility has been achieved, practising nurses may be able to progress along the theory acceptance and application continuum (see Figure 6.1). But how do individual nurses know what stage of this continuum they are currently at, and, if they wish, how do they progress to a more advanced stage? Realising the vital role they can play in applying theory may help.

Involving practitioners has many advantages. Firlit (1990) believes that taking the experiences of practitioners into account is a vital link in establishing a 'theory-practice arena'. Chalmers (1989) argues that it is only by involving clinicians in assessing the worth of theories that a firmer body of practice-related knowledge will be established. Therefore, any discussion about the application of theories must include practice-based staff. This is a valid strategy considering that it is the practitioner who ultimately has to translate the 'know that' of theories into the 'know how' of practice and vice versa. So, the development and field testing of new theories must necessarily involve clinical nurses.

Practising nurses can also identify and reflect on clinical phenomena which can be brought to the attention of nursing in general and theorists in particular. Further, as alluded to above, theorists such as Roper *et al.* (1990), Roy (1980) and Orem (1995) value very

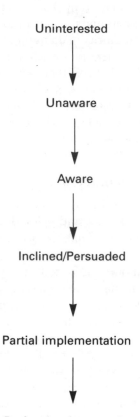

Uninterested

Unaware

Aware

Inclined/Persuaded

Partial implementation

Perfect implementation

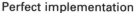

Figure 6.1   Theory acceptance and application continuum
Source: Adapted from Brett (1987)

highly the feedback they received from practitioners concerning
the applicability of their theories.

McKenna (1994a) found in his study that practitioners would
implement theories if they had a better understanding of them. Most
had not been given the time, the opportunity, the support or the
education needed to comprehend theories or realise their potential
for clinical practice. This scenario is not unique to his respondents.

Lerheim (1991) found in her study that it takes time for theories to pass through various filters and for sources to reach practice.

The responsibility, authority and autonomy of the practitioners are other important considerations when trying to apply theories in practice. Vaughan (1990) believes that to introduce a theory nurses have to have the freedom to manage their work and not be bound by the rules and regulations of a rigid hierarchy. Keyzer (1985), whose study has been referred to above, argues for a redistribution of power to patients and ward staff.

The role of nurse managers in theory application

The complex and cumbersome changes in organisation and resources required for the application of nursing theories are generally beyond the capacity of clinically based staff. Managers must allow nurses to question practice and take chances with new theory-based knowledge, and this must be seen as a legitimate use of staff time.

In his research into nursing, Nolan describes the following scenario:

> The manager said that he was all for new ideas but they had to be good ones. Anyone is free to innovate at any time; all they have to do is inform me of what they intend to do and if it is good then they will have my support. Keep in mind that I am sick to death of . . . nurses who think they have wonderful ideas that will change the world.
>
> (Nolan, 1989: 286)

So much for valuing and motivating practitioners. Hunink (1995) describes how staff can be motivated if a nursing policy is based upon a specific nursing theory. However, I think it depends on what form the policy takes. I am aware of several hospitals where management have introduced nursing theories as policies. In two cases the policy states that all patients being admitted to the hospital should be assessed using Roper's theory. This has led to patients who enter hospital for simple procedures, such as the removal of ingrown toenails, being asked by staff about their fears of dying or about expressing sexuality. For nurses not to include these issues in their assessment would be to ignore (at their peril) hospital policy.

The desire to apply nursing theories cannot occur in such collaborative and communication vacuums. It must be incorporated into the organisation's culture rather than being superimposed upon it. Within such a culture, managers should employ the following strategies:

- Support and fund for staff to attend theory conferences;
- Support continuing education in theory awareness;
- Support the formation of theory interest groups and journal clubs;
- Support the formation of 'practice development units' where theory application is foremost;
- support the affiliation of units/wards with university departments;
- Support the setting up of lecturer-practitioner posts whose incumbents can try out new theories through action research approaches;
- Incorporate theory application/awareness into the annual performance review of each staff member.

The involvement of management will be stressed further when planned change is being discussed.

The role of nurse educators in theory application

Throughout the Western world nurse education is moving into universities. At their best, universities are centres where theoretical knowledge is both discovered and transmitted. In those countries in which nursing has been delayed in gaining admission to universities, the development of theoretical knowledge has also been delayed. Practitioners in any discipline are best able to appreciate and apply theory when they have been educated from the beginning in an environment where theory in their field is being generated, challenged and tested, as well as being taught. Nursing and nurse education have some catching up to do – most registered nurse teachers have not received their professional education in such an academic environment. Without such theoretical literacy they will have difficulty instilling the knowledge and skills of theory appreciation, awareness and application in their students.

Gould (1989) warns that if staff on a ward reach consensus on a theory that is not known or taught by the teaching staff, the situation will continue where learners are exposed to one set of practice guides in the classroom and another in the clinical areas. Therefore, one way to encourage the application of theories in the clinical area is for educators to underpin curricula with theories that match practice (Kershaw, 1986). In other words, if a curriculum is structured around a particular nursing theory and the same theory is used by practitioners, then the theory–practice gap could be narrowed for both students and staff.

To encourage students to be critical consumers of theory, a section of most contemporary nursing courses emphasises the importance of nurses being able to critique and analyse theory. This is a laudable objective. However, being able to judge the appropriateness and validity of a theory for practice is not the same as being able or willing actually to use it. In other words, graduates of nursing programmes may be theory-aware, and may be able to critique the commoner theories used, but they may still not be motivated to apply theory to practical situations.

Educators must ensure that this generation and the next generation of nurses are advanced practitioners – basing their practice on sound and relevant theory. Educational programmes on theory appreciation, awareness and application should be the norm, and nurse teachers have a key role to play in the dissemination of up-to-date theoretical information and in producing students who have a realistic critical perception of theory and its uses.

The role of nurse theorists in theory application

Theorists tend to publish in academic journals read mostly by academics and their work is mostly reported at conferences attended by existing theory worshippers. Also, nurse theorists do themselves few favours by overloading their theories with jargon which is confusing for the uninitiated practising nurse and, on top of all this, there are so many theories that it is difficult for any practitioner to make sense of them all! Yet another problem is that theorists often simply publish their work and opt out – believing that an interested practitioner will read their articles and books and implement the theory with their patients. Such practices lead to a time-lag of a number of years between the theory being reported in the literature and being applied in practice. Therefore, there is a frightening prospect that theories could be out of date before they reach patient care level!

Nurse theorists need to be accountable for their work and reduce the time-lag between formulating the theory and presenting it to theory consumers. But are theorists accountable for their work? Will the day arrive when they can be sued if their theory leads to practice which proves to be inappropriate? To avoid this, theorists must provide practising nurses with an understandable theory which includes adequate information about how the theory was developed and tested; but most of all they require a full and helpful discussion of the relevance and potential usefulness of the theory for patient care.

However, as Smoyak (1988) argued, not all theories can be applied in practice, and much of the theory that can is at the descriptive and explanatory level rather than at the prescriptive level. There has been a tendency for nurse theorists to concentrate on grand theories which avoid those practice issues which have immense importance for the well-being of patients. Perhaps there would be an increase in the use of theories if more were formulated at mid-range and practice theory level. Such theories can make a substantial contribution to nursing interventions and their outcomes.

There is also a body of opinion that believes nurses cannot afford to compartmentalise themselves totally as unidisciplinary theorists but must be involved in theorising with multidisciplinary colleagues (Meleis, 1991). While this may be a long-term goal, in the interim, more theorising in partnership with practising nurses and patients is also a definite way forward. To paraphrase Orr (1992), theorists would then be extending their role from being generators of new knowledge to being enhancers of knowledge-generating capacities in practitioners.

Planned change for theory-based practice

There is much confusion in the literature between the terms 'change' and 'innovation'. Change may be defined as an attempt to alter or replace existing knowledge, skills, attitudes, norms and styles of individuals and groups (Wright, 1988: 154). On the other hand, innovations in nursing imply changes in practice that are new to those using them and that are intended to benefit clients (Haller, Reynolds and Horsley, 1979: 46). So innovation is change, but with the added implication of novelty and newness.

Types of change

Leddy and Pepper (1989) identified four types of change. These are 'haphazard', 'spontaneous', 'developmental' and 'planned'. All these types of change have been used at one time or another to introduce theories into clinical practice. Haphazard change is generally random and unpredictable. It is impossible to anticipate when it will take place and participants are never prepared for its arrival. Spontaneous change is also unpredictable and unanticipated but it tends to occur as a response to natural events. Developmental change is related to growth and takes the form of sequential orderly phases and is mostly predictable and controllable. Planned change is deliberate and carried out with conscious intent.

According to Sampson (1971: 226), a social psychologist, planned change is an intentional effort to intervene in an ongoing state in order to produce a new state. Rogers (1983. 6) has a more comprehensive view, believing that planned change is a process by which new ideas are created or developed (invention), communicated to all participants (diffusion) and either adopted or rejected (consequences).

Theories of change

Within the social sciences there are many theories and taxonomies of change. It is proposed to give a brief overview of the work of some of the major change theorists. Perhaps the best known is Kurt Lewin (1951).

Lewin's theory of change

Lewin's theory posits the idea of a force field involving protagonists of and antagonists to change. For change to occur there must be an upset in the equilibrium between these two forces. He identified three basic steps for introducing planned change. These are unfreezing, moving and refreezing.

Unfreezing involves a destabilising of the forces that are preserving the status quo. The organisation is ready for unfreezing if expectations have not been met, if there is guilt or anxiety owing to some action or lack of action and if previous obstacles to change have disappeared. Lewin believes that unfreezing can be accomplished by provisional involvement, direct confrontation, acceptance of ambivalence and by the creation of a vacuum. These strategies will instil in participants the need for change and the motivation to change.

In the second step, moving, the change is implemented and 'cognitive redefinition' takes place among those involved in the change process. Cognitive redefinition involves viewing the situation from a different perspective. This can occur through 'identification' or 'scanning'. In identification, the participants are influenced towards change by someone who has power or their respect. In scanning, the participants review the possibilities and select the best approach by mutual decision. The status quo is then left behind and the organisation moves to a new level of functioning. Refreezing, the last step in Lewin's theory, involves the introduction of stability and equilibrium at the new level. The new method of work or behaviour is then internalised into the culture of the organisation and into the actions of participants.

Many subsequent change theorists believe that Lewin's theory is not intricate enough to deal with all the complexities of planned change. As a result, Schein (1969), Lippitt (1973) and Rogers (1983) have used Lewin's theory as a foundation for more comprehensive theories of change.

Resistance to change

Fretwell (1985) gives a very useful overview of the literature on change. She shows that health care settings are particularly resistant to change, and, where change is initiated, it is often short-lived. Nurses also appear to be resistant to change. According to Adam (1983), the prospect of giving up a certain way of being a nurse and substituting a more precise way is a frightening and dangerous proposal since there is no guarantee that the end result will be to everyone's entire satisfaction. Not all nurses are willing to take the risk; some are even convinced that there is no risk involved in avoiding change (1983: 78).

Lindsay (1990) asserts that nursing is still deeply traditional and suspicious of innovations. This assertion is not surprising if we agree with Salvage's view (1990: 3) that change in nursing is usually drawn out, painful, messy and unfair. Many other writers have tried to identify reasons for resistance to change. One reason may be the lack of reward given to practising nurses who show evidence of creativity and innovation. While health service managers get performance-related pay for introducing change, there is no economic inducement for nurses to change their practices. Other reasons for resistance to change include an affection for the established order of things, insufficient time, reluctance to admit lack of knowledge, the imposition of change by power and coercion, powerlessness within the change process, lack of ownership of the change and the negative views of their powerful multidisciplinary colleagues. There are also psychological reasons for resistance to change such as insecurity, fear of the unknown, fear of failure and fear of loosing power and prestige (Leddy and Pepper, 1989).

From the above it can be seen that there is a strong link between change and feelings of anxiety. Moreover, there is early research evidence that nursing is an anxiety-provoking occupation (Menzies, 1960). Acknowledging this evidence, Fretwell (1985) postulates that during a process of change nurses may experience greater levels of anxiety and 'future shock' than members of other occupations. Future shock has been defined as the shattering stress and disorientation that we induce in individuals by subjecting them to too much stress in too short a time (Toffler, 1970: 4).

A review of the literature in social psychology offers other views on possible reasons for resistance to change. Seligman (1971) described 'learned helplessness' where individuals feel they have little or no control over the outcome of their actions. Earlier, Rotter (1966) wrote of the importance of 'locus of control'; individuals must have a certain amount of control over the changes that affect their practices. The effect of locus of control on resistance is highlighted by

Rogers (1974: 360) who stated that resistance may be expected when one feels pressured to make a change and will be decreased when one has a say in the nature or direction of the change.

Watson (1973) identifies five stages in resistance to change. In the first stage, resistance is very great and undifferentiated. In the second stage, the antagonists and protagonists for change can be identified. In the third stage, resistance is mobilised to undermine the proposed change. In the fourth stage, the protagonists are more powerful and the antagonists are seen as mere nuisances. In the fifth and final stage, the antagonists are very much in the minority and have little influence on the change.

Six different types of participant have been identified based upon their readiness to resist change (Rogers, 1983). These are the 'innovators' who are normally well motivated and eager for change. The 'early adopters' express moderate enthusiasm for the proposed change. The 'early majority adopters' seldom take the lead in changing practices but they are open to change. The 'late majority adopters' are cynical about change and require peer group pressure. The 'laggards', as supporters of the status quo, are suspicious and active in their resistance to change. The 'rejectors' openly resist the change and may try to sabotage it by discouraging others.

Change strategies

Chin and Benne (1976) maintain that to keep resistance to change at a minimum and to facilitate successful change it is important to select an appropriate change strategy. They identified three main strategies. These are the 'empirical-rational' strategy, the 'normative-re-educative' strategy and the 'power-coercive' strategy.

The empirical-rational change strategy

This strategy is based on the assumption that people are rational beings and will always be logical in their actions, especially if it is in their own interests to be so. Therefore, it is assumed that if nurses are given in-service education on the merits of a proposed innovation they will willingly adopt the change. According to Lancaster and Lancaster (1982), when this strategy is successful the change is fast, efficient and long lasting. However, this strategy may not always be successful. For instance, although research has found smoking, eating fatty foods and practising unprotected sex with multiple partners to be detrimental to health, rational individuals still carry out these practices. Therefore, the reasonable logical argument is not always a stimulus to change.

The normative-re-educative change strategy

This strategy also assumes that the participants in the change process are rational beings. However, an added dimension is the emphasis on the change of attitudes and values. Group work is an important part of this strategy and ownership of the change by the group members is emphasised. When successful, this strategy encourages commitment from the participants, but it often takes longer to accomplish compared to the other two strategies.

The power-coercive change strategy

This strategy is normally a 'top-down' initiative and depends on the use of power. The participants are not normally involved in the planning of the proposed change but must accept its imposition. Of the three strategies, this is the fastest way of implementing change, but it seldom lasts very long. Notwithstanding this, Leddy and Pepper (1989) argue that, regardless of whether knowledge or attitudes are modified, change will only occur when it is supported by power.

Perhaps, in a situation where change to theory-based practice is required, there is room for all three of these strategies. Hersey and Blanchard (1977) outline only two change strategies: 'participative' and 'coercive'. The former is similar to the empirical-rational and the normative-re-educative approaches, while the latter coincides with the power-coercive strategy. Zaltman and Duncan (1977) group strategies for change into four categories. These are 're-education', 'persuasion', 'power' and 'facilitation'. These categories also broadly coincide with Chin and Benne's (1976) work.

Failure of change

Readers may wonder why, after introducing nursing theories into practice, nurses lose interest in them with such speed. Having examined the implementation of organisational change in the National Health Service, Moscow (1986) notes that failure to sustain change was normally owing to one or more of the factors identified in Box 6.1. Time and difficulty are important variables to consider when planning a change to theory-based practice. Hersey and Blanchard's (1977) framework has been adapted to illustrate these issues with regard to theory application. It can be seen from Figure 6.2 that a change in knowledge about nursing theories would be relatively easy to obtain in a short time frame. A change in attitudes takes a little longer and is more difficult to achieve. A change by an individual to theory-based practice is more difficult and is time-consuming to achieve. Finally, a change where all staff are enthusiastically using the theory is very difficult and is the most time-consuming of all.

Box 6.1 Factors contributing to a failure to sustain change

- incomplete diagnosis;
- starting off too fast;
- missionary zeal for the 'flavour of the month';
- losing the senior sponsor;
- lack of steering from the steering group;
- proceeding too fast for people to absorb the consequences;
- demands for unrealistic short-term results;
- failing to evaluate benefits as they occur;
- not monitoring the boundaries;
- failing to get 'key players' in the right state of commitment and support;
- insufficient involvement of the people affected by the changes;
- insufficient resources allocated to maintain the change.

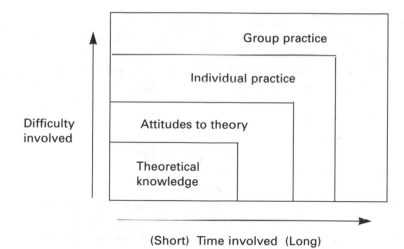

Figure 6.2   Change to theory-based practice in terms of time and difficulty

The change process in applying nursing theories

Salanders and Dietz-Omar (1991) found that the introduction of a nursing theory represented a change in the philosophical orientation of the nurse. Earlier, Wright (1988) had argued that change will occur in any setting where a nursing theory is being adopted. On the authority of Robinson (1990), the adoption of a nursing theory is essentially a precursor to radical change. It is an explicit call to change practice. That is why, of course, so many of the proponents of the use of theories in practice are those who are at the forefront of change. They care about the nursing practice they offer and are constantly seeking ways to improve it (1990: 11).

Therefore, it is not surprising that the literature dealing with the introduction of nursing theories into clinical practice tends to follow the various theories and strategies of change outlined above. However, Robinson's view can only be accepted with certain reservations. I am of the opinion that, without proper understanding and planning, the adoption of theory-based practice will not be a precursor to radical change.

Assessing the need for a nursing theory in practice

Applying a nursing theory to practice is a task that should only be undertaken after much preparation. Prior to its introduction, it is important to make sure that the theory is not going to replace a more appropriate one already in use. Therefore, it is essential to find out how good or bad the existing formal or informal theory is.

Most of the literature stresses that the introduction of a nursing theory requires considerable time, dedication, commitment and support, both moral and financial (Jones, 1990). Efforts have to be made to ensure that all those who are going to be affected by the theory, including nurses, patients, their families and multidisciplinary colleagues, understand its philosophy and find it acceptable.

It may also be prudent to assess the attitudes of clinical staff and patients towards nursing theories and towards change in general. Sharp (1991) states that attitudes are precursors of behaviour and a person's attitude may constitute a predisposition to respond to something in a negative or positive way. So, a negative attitude towards nursing theories and an unwillingness to change will influence the motivation to change and the acceptance of the change.

Careful assessment of the environment is also important, as ward layout can sometimes thwart attempts to implement a nursing theory successfully (Aggleton and Chalmers, 1990). However, the resources required to make the environment more receptive to theory-based practice may be difficult to obtain when there are increasing financial restraints and when existing services are stretched to the limit.

Capers (1986) summarised the major assessments that must be made prior to introducing a nursing theory. She believes it is important to determine whether the nursing practice environment is conducive to using the nursing theory, what outcomes are anticipated for its use, which nursing personnel will use the theory, how staff are to be prepared to use the theory, how and when the theory will be evaluated and what financial resources are needed compared to what is available (cited in Fawcett, 1989: 54).

Planning the change to theory-based practice

According to Wright (1988), the power-coercive approach is not an appropriate change strategy for the implementation of a nursing theory. If this is attempted, he warns that a 'shifting sands effect' will occur, with a reversion to old norms once the initiator of the change moves on. He advocates a 'bottom-up' normative-re-educative approach with active involvement of clinical nurses.

When planning change it is important to have a collaborative approach with all those affected being involved in the discussions. In their study into the use of Orem's theory, Denyes *et al.* (1989) found that communication was critical to the success of the venture. Frequent meetings of interested parties enhanced mutual understanding of the goals, plans, methods, problems and solutions. Discussions among participants were especially valuable for standardising the implementation approach. Chapman (1990: 14) also stresses the importance of communications, believing that the ethical way to introduce a nursing theory is to hold discussions with clinical nurses, managers and nurse educators so that they can decide for themselves whether a particular nursing theory merits experimental implementation.

Implementing the change to theory-based practice

Some writers place the responsibility of implementing a nursing theory solely in the hands of practitioners (McFarlane, 1986a; Luker, 1987). However, others suggest (as with the assessment and planning phases) a co-ordinated approach involving management, teachers and clinical staff working together over a substantial period (Walsh, 1990). The latter approach involves group situations that enable the staff to come together for mutual support and for democratic discussions on implementation problems. One way forward is to introduce a nursing theory using a pilot group of patients. This decreases the amount of 'future shock' and also focuses the contributions of the practitioners involved.

Salanders and Dietz-Omar (1991) maintain that the first major step in implementing a nursing theory is to have formal and informal educational sessions. This will help the ward staff to become familiar with the theory and give them the skills necessary to apply it. According to Dyer (1990), this will make it meaningful to them and help to minimise their fears and anxieties about the new theory.

As referred to in the previous chapter, the theory may have to be adapted to suit particular patient care problems and care planning documentation will have to be changed. When using the nursing process to apply a theory, Kershaw and Salvage (1986) stress the difficulty of nurses identifying patients' needs that cannot be met. They suggest that it is more realistic for the assessment to be directed solely and specifically to those patient needs that the nurse is able to meet through a constructive and achievable care plan (1986: xiii).

Critics of nursing theories argue that, in most areas where nursing theories are introduced, the change is superficial and old practices endure. Fretwell (1985) states that nurses become adept at producing a veneer of change through documentation while leaving underlying practices untouched. In the words of Vaughan (1990), 'the change is only skin deep'. Therefore, although suitable documentation is important, the theory's philosophy must be reflected in the culture of the setting and the care carried out with patients.

Evaluating the change to theory-based practice

The dearth of research literature on the evaluation of theories in practice has already been alluded to in the previous chapter. Researchers like Denyes *et al.* (1989) give some guidance on what should be evaluated. They support Suchman's (1967) process-outcome approach to evaluation. However, Walsh (1990) acknowledges that, prior to doing this, reliable and valid tools must be formulated. He states that just measuring patient satisfaction is no longer appropriate.

In conclusion, there is a wealth of literature which suggests that theory-based practice can make a substantial contribution to patient care. While this is laudable, if an applied theory is not having positive effects on the thinking and behaviour of staff and the outcomes of patients, like food that has passed its sell-by date it should be discarded before it does harm.

Summary

There is much confusion and many conflicting ideas in the literature regarding the application of nursing theories to client care.

Some authors maintain that theories must be relevant for practice, while others suggest that many theories were not meant for direct implementation with clients at all; rather, theories stimulate thinking and reflection among practitioners. Nevertheless, throughout the UK, nurses are attempting to use them in practice. Many stress that these theories will strengthen the link between the classroom and the clinical areas, hence bridging the theory–practice gap. However, others argue that theories can only perpetuate this divide.

Although there are wide-ranging opinions, there is a dearth of sound research studies available which have examined how nursing theories affect client care. More studies need to be done and those few which have been done require replication. The use of methods such as action research, phenomenology and quasi-experiments to note the results of implementing theories must be seen as a legitimate use of research funding and researchers' time.

From the research that does exist, it would appear that to look favourably on the utilisation of theory is to look favourably on quality of care. It could be argued that one nurse applying theory to improve the quality of client care is of more value than dozens of nurses developing theories which are not tested and will never be applied in practice. This may appear to some to be heretical, but the mere existence of theories cannot alter client care; they have to be used to be effective.

Chapter 7
Theory and research: the relationship

In Chapter 6, the close association between theory and practice was explored. This was envisaged as a reciprocal relationship where theory can grow from practice and be returned to guide practice. This chapter introduces you to a third partner in this process, namely, research.

Jacox (1974), reflecting on the relationship between theory and research, stated that research without theory was analogous to a team of bricklayers, each making a brick in isolation from other bricklayers and with no blueprint to follow. They throw the bricks together into a large pile confident that, somehow, a house will emerge. Without theory, therefore, nursing knowledge would be a mass of data, statistics and observations with no coherence or understanding (Moody, 1990).

Knowledge is of little use without understanding. Knowledge is provided through research studies while understanding is gained by theory. It is a reciprocal relationship; while knowledge can increase in nursing for a time without understanding, understanding is not possible without new knowledge being developed. According to Lorraine Walker (1971), the result of theory being unable to keep pace with knowledge development is stagnation of the discipline.

Practice should lead to theory, theory should lead to research, and research should lead back to practice. In other words, new theory generated from practice will lead to new studies which will lead to new knowledge for practice, and new knowledge presents us with new facts which encourages us to develop theories to explain these facts. Unfortunately, within nursing this tripartite interacting structure of theory, research and practice does not always function as a unit. Too often, practice is carried out without being guided by research or theory. Similarly, much of the research in nursing has been descriptive and poorly linked to theory, and studies continue to be undertaken without cognisance of any theoretical alliance.

Research is a tool of science and its function is enquiry. The product of science is theory and these theories go to make up the working parts of our body of knowledge for practice. Science craves an understanding of phenomena through creating some unifying or organising frameworks about the nature of these phenomena (theory generation) and science evaluates these frameworks for their empirical honesty (theory testing).

Meleis (1991) states that researchers view theorists as 'ivory tower' philosophers who dream up ideas unconnected with practice or research. Theorists view researchers as investigators who focus on small research projects using a foreign positivist approach to confirm or not confirm disconnected propositions that do not add up to theory.

Completing isolated non-cumulative research projects that do not lead to development or corroboration of theories has limited usefulness. Further, the end product of research is poor if it does not provide theoretical formulations for the explanation of phenomena, prediction of events, situations or responses or for the prescription of interventions. Kuhn (1970) argues that this is indicative of a discipline at a preparadigmatic stage of development.

Previously, Dickoff and James (1968) called for theory-linked research. They stated that research is for the sake of theory and theory is for the sake of practice, and that theory produced without research has little hope of viability. Using the metaphor of metallurgy they likened research to an assaying tool that tests presented materials in the light of their claims. They also use the metaphor of the divining-rod, where research can point to areas worthy of further digging because of sensed promise. Research, they say, is pointless unless done (a) in the context of theory and (b) with a clear realisation of what it can contribute to theory.

In 1964, Brown urged nurse researchers to ask themselves the following questions:

● In what ways and to what extent is this investigation linked to theory?

- What contributions does this investigation make to a scientific body of knowledge?
- Is the theoretical framework from one of the basic sciences an applied science or more specifically nursing theory?

She proceeded to state that a theoretical base of science not deeply rooted in rigorously conducted research could suffer from erroneous fabrication by 'armchair theorists' or could misdirect practitioners and educators into using faulty knowledge. Most grand theories in nursing were developed as 'armchair theories'; there is nothing wrong with this, while theorists accepted only the first part of Cartesian rationalism – they generated the theory by reasoning and reflection, but did not bother to test it.

Brown appears to find it unacceptable that the theoretical formulations of 'armchair theorists' may be useful. However, she does not acknowledge the fact that theory may exist before the research is undertaken to test it. Supporting Brown's stance, Walker (1971) warns that if nurses are taught theories which have little or no research support, the nursing care based on these theories may have detrimental effects on clients. She argues that while nursing actions based on theory which has not been validated may be creative and may give security to nurses, they remain in the realm of myth and non-scientific knowledge. Walker suggests that there are serious ethical implications for such practices.

Both these authors do have valid arguments. However, I believe that in so far as they may stretch our view of nursing and push forward the boundaries of our thinking, untested theories may be a welcome addition to our theoretical repertoire. None the less, I have to accept that their implementation in practice in an unquestioning manner may do a great deal of harm and may become just as much a ritual as the habitual carrying out of existing nursing practices.

In nursing, theory and research have been divided into two camps. First, there are hypothesis-testing studies where, through deductive testing, the object is to create predictive and practice theories (situation-relating and situation-producing theories, see Chapter 4). Such research has been labelled 'positivism', 'empiricism' or 'quantitative research', where observation and measurable behaviour are seen as more scientific than the accompanying thought processes. Qualitative research makes up the second camp where, through inductive development, the object is to create descriptive and explanatory theories. Such research has been labelled 'soft science' and has been berated by empiricists as being unduly subjective.

Chalmers (1989) points out that positivist approaches to theory development mimic work in the natural sciences where researchers are motivated to discover universal laws. In nursing this may be a fruitless search, for, considering our proposed sensitivity to the individuality of human beings, such laws may be untenable. In contrast, qualitative researchers are less likely to search for causal relationships and theories which have universal application. According to Field and Morse (1985) it is the place of theory in the research process which distinguishes quantitative from qualitative approaches. Qualitative inductive approaches focus on careful in-depth examination of data to look for patterns and hypotheses which may then be developed and tested in order to generate theory. Alternatively, quantitative deductive approaches identify existing theory, formulate hypotheses from propositions, identify variables, collect data, do statistical analysis and check if the theory has been refuted or supported.

Fawcett and Downs (1992) agree with this distinction. In keeping with a post-positivist perspective they argue that all observation is theory laden. They assert that research does one of two things: it generates theory or it tests theory. In theory generating research the investigator seeks to identify a phenomenon, discover its dimensions or characteristics, or specify the relationships between the dimensions; in theory testing research the investigator seeks to develop evidence about hypotheses derived from theory.

Stevens-Barnum (1994) is another metatheorist who does not recognise the existence of research which is not linked in some way to theory. She maintains that theory directs research, research corrects theory, and corrected theory directs more research.

In contrast, Chinn and Kramer (1995) argue that there are two main types of research: 'theory-linked research' and 'theory-isolated research'. They concede that both can be of excellent quality and can contribute to new knowledge but, because the former is conducted within the framework of theory, it has greater potential for developing new knowledge. Theory-linked research is related to the generation or the testing of theory while theory-isolated research has no discernible theoretical connection. In both types of research, questions may come from the imagination, from work experience, from a hunch or a number of other sources. The findings from theory-linked research can be retranslated to theoretic terms and implications discussed in relation to the theory.

Linkages between research and theory

Accepting what these various authors have said, in my experience there are four linkages between research and theory:

- Research tests theory deductively in practice (theory-testing research or TTR);
- Research generates theory inductively from practice (theory-generating research or TGR);
- Theory guides the research project (theory-framed research or TFR);
- Research evaluates the use of theory in practice (theory-evaluating research or TER).

Theory-testing research (TTR)

Because those who undertake TTR propose an a priori construction of theory from which prepositional and hypothetical statements are derived and then verified or falsified through research, TTR could be referred to as the 'theory-then-research' process.

Put simply, in TTR a theory exists and research is undertaken to establish its validity. The research methods in theory-testing studies are designed to ascertain how accurately the theory depicts real-world phenomena and their relationships. It has to be stressed that an entire theory is not tested by one study; rather, concepts and propositions from that theory are isolated in some manner in order to be tested. Empirical indicators of the relevant concepts must be used. Within grand theory, not all concepts have empirical indicators and this is another reason why only parts of a theory can be tested.

According to Chinn and Kramer (1995) for a theory to be testable you need:

- Concepts that describe the empirical world;
- Theoretical and operational definitions of concepts;
- Constructs and propositions;
- Links among the concepts and constructs that explain or predict phenomena.

As mentioned above, theory testing normally involves a deductive approach whereby hypotheses are tested using randomised controlled trials, experimental or quasi-experimental approaches. Research questions can also be used in theory testing – this usually takes place within a correlational design. The concepts within the research questions or hypotheses are derived from the theory and the findings have implications for the theory. Figure 7.1 shows one such theory-testing process. This process is not necessarily linear, it may be iterative. For TTR to be robust, there must be consistency and congruency between the conceptual reasoning and the study design, its conduct and the interpretation of result.

Writing up the report

In TTR the research purpose, the research problem and the hypotheses/research questions are designed to show the relationships between the theory and the research study, and these are formulated in advance of conducting the investigation. Previous studies based upon the theory form a substantial part of the literature review. The review also includes a critique of research based on alternative theories and/or concepts shown to be relevant to the study's central purpose. Further, the literature review indicates how the study was conceived and why the specific relationships within the theory are being tested. There is also a critical discussion of existing research that supports or refutes the theoretical assertions as well as the theoretical basis for the hypotheses or research questions (Fawcett and Downs, 1992).

In TTR the data are collected by direct (physical) observation or indirect (interviews and self-completion tools) observation. The reliability and validity of the data-collection tools are given serious

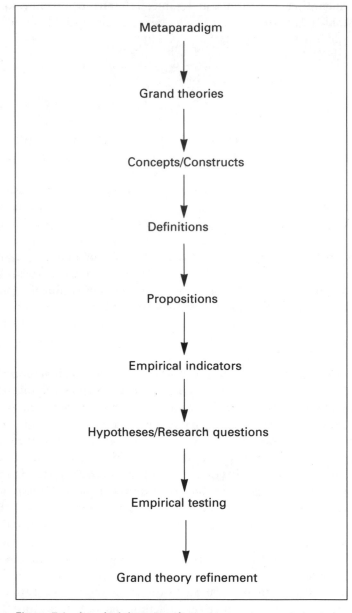

Figure 7.1   A typical theory-testing process
adapted from Moody, 1990

consideration. The sample and population must be carefully considered and invariably statistical power analysis is used in deciding the sample size. The researcher may manipulate the independent variable with an experimental group to note what effect it has on specific dependent variables. In TTR the analysis focuses on whether the data present sufficient quantitative (or qualitative) evidence to support or reject the hypotheses or answer the research questions. In the discussion section of the study, conclusions are made regarding the empirical adequacy of the theory.

In TTR, the findings may:

- Support the validity of the theory;
- Refute the validity of the theory;
- Lead to the theory being adapted or revised;
- Lead to the formulation of a new theory.

The reasons why a theory is supported or refuted may not always be obvious, but knowledge has been expanded and possible false leads have been eradicated (Stevens-Barnum, 1994). Readers may be intrigued by the idea that theory-testing research may actually lead to theory generation. Strange as it may seem, because of the insight gained through the research, the basis for a new theory may be formed!

However, Stevens-Barnum (1994: 272) warns that those seeking eternal truths should not rely on TTR. She supports her warning with the following research hypothesis: 'if theory X is true then consequences Q, R, S will follow under conditions A and B.' One then tests the theory to see if this happens and, if it does, then the theory is confirmed. But later some other person may present a better or equally good explanation as to why the consequences occurred under those conditions. Therefore, a theory is the accepted explanation for phenomena only until a better theory comes along.

Sorenson (1986, cited in Moody, 1990) argued that nursing must:

- Develop innovative strategies for theory testing through research;
- Encourage nurse scholars to generate testable hypotheses deduced from the underlying assumptions and propositions of existing nursing theories;

- Organise multiple site studies at national and international levels where several investigators can focus on systematic testing of hypotheses from nursing theories;
- Identify criteria for theory testing in nursing research and nursing theory courses;
- Collaborate in national and international research endeavours with practitioners who are engaged in implementing nursing theories in clinical areas.

However, some theories are not testable because of ethical considerations. For instance, while theories may be formulated on starvation among babies or on mother–child separation, it would be unethical to test them in practice. There are other reasons for theories not being testable. Stevens-Barnum (1994) reminds us that the subject-matter may be too abstract or the methods required to test the theory may not (as yet) exist. The technology and methods required to test Einstein's theory of relativity ($E=MC^2$) were not available until many years after it was developed.

As mentioned in the introduction, the 'hypothetico/deductive' TTR method is congruent with the traditional positivist/empirical science approach to knowledge development. Here, measurement is extremely important. Over twenty-five years ago Rosemary Ellis (1970) asserted that if nurse researchers limited themselves to that which can be measured, they ran the risk of studying trivia or issues tangential to nursing. She feared that too much reliance on quantification would lead to premature closure and that an adherence to the ideals of an empirical design could be constraining for a developing discipline. More recently, Sarter (1988) pointed out that all events are subject to interpretation and that theorists also interpret events when theorising. If we accept this, then interpretative qualitative approaches should be used to test the validity of theory. From a scientific and knowledge development standpoint, Sarter and Ellis are not isolated in their thinking. The arch-rationalist Karl Popper (1965) admitted that the verification of theory involves intuition.

To conclude this section: there has been a great deal written about the necessity of testing nursing theories to provide evidence of the validity and accuracy of their concepts and assumptions.

However, little progress has been made towards this goal either by the theorists themselves, by researchers or by those nurses who use them in practice. Dickoff and James (1968) recommend such testing, claiming that not to do so would have consequences for the quality of care. This is understandable considering the implications of nurses using a model of dubious validity as an organising framework for the care of patients.

An overview of the literature on theory testing in nursing is presented in Chapter 8 as part of theory analysis and evaluation. Readers will note that within the literature what is meant by 'theory testing' is not often made clear, and in fact few authors are in agreement as to how it should be undertaken.

Theory-generating research (TGR)

To date, most of the research in nursing has been of the theory-testing variety with little concern for where and how theories were developed. Speaking generally for science, Laudan (1977) stated that theoretical progress in a discipline is measured to a great extent by the number and the quality of the theories developed by its scholars. Speaking specifically for nursing, Brown (1964) stated that the most useful measure of research outcome is the growth in sound theory on which to base nursing care and education. Here, Brown is stressing that a key function of research is to generate theory.

When little is known about the phenomena, TGR research is conducted for the purpose of discovery and exploration of the phenomena as they occur in the natural world. The resultant theories are normally generated inductively by researchers who realise that nursing practice constitutes the phenomenological field for the observation and collection of data. Because the research eventually leads to inductively formulated theory, TGR may be referred to as the 'research-then-theory' approach to knowledge development.

Supporting the clinical setting as the basis for theory, Dickoff and James (1992) claim that, since nursing practice predates nursing research, it makes a sound foundation for theorising rather than theory being built up through research that is purposefully isolated from practice. Furthermore, if nurse researchers are to be major developers of theoretical knowledge, they must work in partnership with clinical staff who can provide them with research worthy topics concerning the phenomena of specific interest to patient care.

Chinn and Kramer (1995) point out that, when attempting to generate theory, the researcher enters the research setting with as open a mind as possible in order to see new relationships between concepts. Because we all have our own conceptual baggage which we bring to new situations, this is not always an easy process. Therefore, while 'bracketing out' all previous experience is impossible, we should be acutely aware of our possible biases.

Theory can be generated both through interpretative qualitative studies and empirical quantitative studies. There follows a brief overview of the approaches favoured by these two schools. I would refer the reader to Chapter 2 for a more in-depth exploration of the philosophy underpinning these approaches and to a research textbook if they seek more detailed information regarding the research methodology.

Interpretative qualitative approaches to theory generation

Grounded theory approach: this involves the simultaneous collection of data, coding, categorising observations and forming concepts and relationships based on the data. In grounded theory the researcher begins to write impressions about the meaning of the data as they are collected (Glaser and Strauss, 1967).

Ethnography: this approach has its basis in social anthropology. The researcher seeks to get involved in the setting, and soak up the concepts which are important in describing that situation.

Non-participant observation: this approach collects rich data about phenomena using a 'fly-on-the-wall' type methodology.

Phenomenology: this is designed to describe the subjective lived experiences of people and to comprehend the essence and meanings that people place on these experiences. The experiences cannot be observed, they can only be directly accessible to the person who has the experience. Through interviewing or using unstructured questionnaires people can describe how they felt or how they remember certain situations.

Phenomenology results in narratives where the participant has told his or her story about his or her lived experience. Grounded theory results in new or existing concepts joined together by propositional statements. Both ethnography and non-participant observation result in observations that, when examined, lead to new ways of viewing phenomena. Regardless of approach, findings are usually presented in the form of concepts and propositions which form the basis for a new theory. While the end result of TGR is often mid-range theory the following grand theories were developed using interpretative qualitative approaches: Patterson and Zderad (1976), Parse (1981), Benner (1984) and Watson (1985).

Empirical quantitative approaches to theory generation

Jacox (1974) identified three empiricist type stages to the inductive generation of theory.

1 The researcher must identify the phenomena of interest within the field of study and specify, define and classify the concepts used in describing these phenomena;
2 The researcher develops statements or propositions that propose how two or more concepts are related;
3 The researcher specifies how the propositions are related to each other in a systematic way.

The above approaches represent two different philosophical schools of science. None the less, there are similarities in their approach to theory generation. In both cases the source of theory is practice and inductive methods are used. Furthermore, the starting-point in both cases is the phenomena within practice and the end-point is propositional statements forming a new theory.

In the past, emphasis on the empiricist approach alone led to the denigration of those theories which were not formulated in this way, and it caused theorists to distort their theoretical work to fit this approach. Readers must remember that a group supporting one approach will find it easy to criticise the theories generated using the other approach.

Writing up the report

In TGR, the clinical problem, the research problems and the research purpose need to be stated in advance. According to Chinn and Kramer (1995), research hypotheses may also be used. However, more commonly, research questions or problem statements are enough to guide the investigation and hypotheses may be introduced only at the conclusion of the study.

A literature review is not normally completed in advance for, as ideas arise from the data, they guide the researcher in exploring the literature. The review includes the theoretic, philosophic and empiric studies pertinent to the area of concern. There must also be an emphasis on the lack of theory in the area and the theoretical significance of the proposed study should be made explicit at the outset.

In TGR the data are collected by directly (physical observation) or indirectly (unstructured interview schedules). In addition, because of their inherent theoretical bias, research instruments commonly used to collect data in TTR may not be very useful in TGR. Where the aim is to collect narrative data, care must be taken to ensure that the approaches used will elicit the types of response which are required.

Because the sample must link the theoretical aspects of the study to the reality of practice the following assumption is made: there is some phenomenon or event happening in reality that will be evident if I observe these events or this particular group of people. Furthermore, this event or group of people is sufficiently like other events or groups of people who have this experience.

Strange as it may seem, a time series with comparison group can also be used for the qualitative generation of theory. For example, if researchers were studying the experiences of hospitalisation of persons with mental health problems, they might take a longitudinal approach whereby qualitative data are collected before, during and after the hospitalisation. At the same time they might identify other groups of patients with similar problems who are being treated in the community. The comparison would tell the researcher if aspects of the phenomena of anxiety and self-esteem were unique to one type of care or another. These data would contribute to the development of theory related to the hospitalisation experience.

In TGR the analysis of data involves identifying themes and categories which emanate from the data. However, according to Chinn and Kramer (1995), a quantitative, statistical analysis may also be used. Either way, the researcher proposes concepts generated from the data and, if the evidence supports them, theoretical propositions. In most TGR reports the concepts and propositions may not be evident until the results of the data analysis are presented.

As with TTR, the discussion and conclusions focus on the theoretical significance of the study. In TGR, though, the conclusions centre around the newly discovered concepts and relevant propositions. These are often immediately useful in practice because of their grounding in the experience or setting from which the theory is generated. I would refer you to Chapter 3 for a detailed description of propositions. Box 7.1 summarises the types of proposition that may emanate from TGR. According to Fawcett and Downs (1992), the arrangement of propositions in a TGR research report may be easier if they are allocated to groups (e.g., propositions that deal with concept x are put into one group and those relating to concept y into another, and so on) and hierarchically ordered in terms of their level of abstraction.

The next step in TGR is diagramming or putting the concepts and propositions into diagrammatic form. Diagramming is done after the concepts, definitions and propositions have been identified and propositions have been hierarchically ordered by level of abstraction (Fawcett and Downs, 1992). Within the diagram the existence of a relationship is denoted by an unbroken line. For connecting concepts, an arrowhead at one end indicates an asymmetrical relationship and an arrowhead at both ends indicates a symmetrical relationship. A positive relationship is denoted by a + sign and a negative relationship is denoted by a – sign. A question mark may be used if the direction is unclear (see Figure 7.2). Therefore, in a good TGR report the reader is presented with information on the literature pertaining to the phenomenon being

Box 7.1 Types of propositional statement developed through TGR

- Existence of a relationship: there is a relationship between x and y.
- Direction of a relationship: there is a positive relationship between x and y.
- Shape of a relationship: there is a linear relationship between x and y.
- Strength of a relationship: there is a large relationship between x and y.
- Concurrent relationships: if x, then also y.
- Sequential relationships: if x, then later y.
- Deterministic relationships: if x, then always y, if no interfering conditions.
- Probalistic (stochastic) relationships: if x, then probably y.
- Necessary relationships: if x, and only if x, then y.
- Substitutional relationships: if x^1, but also x^2, then y.
- Sufficient relationships: if x, then y, regardless of anything else.
- Contingent relationships: if x, then y, in the presence of c.

studied, on the method employed and on the resultant concepts and propositional statements. Where possible, the researcher should also make clear to the reader what types of propositional statement have been generated and, by diagramming, the relationship is clarified in terms of existence, direction and symmetry. Some of the above propositions may also be stated in terms of testable hypotheses. In this way TGR is opening an opportunity for future TTR to take place (see Figure 7.3).

In TGR, the findings may:

- Lead to the formulation of a new theory;
- Lead to supporting an existing theory;
- Lead to a rejection of an existing theory;
- Lead to an existing theory being adapted or revised.

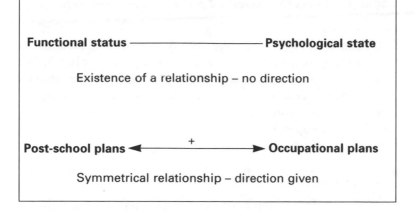

Figure 7.2   Examples of propositional diagramming

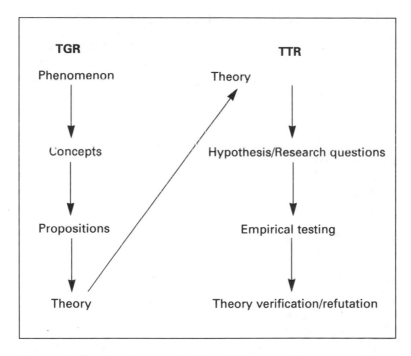

Figure 7.3   The developmental relationship between theory generation and theory testing

Theory-framed research (TFR)

While it is argued that some research does not need theory (Chinn and Kramer, 1995), I believe that all questions asked by a researcher originate in a theoretical framework (whether or not the researcher realises it). Examining qualitative research, Sandelowski (1993) argues forcefully that theory permeates through every aspect of a qualitative research study.

Polit and Hungler (1983) suggest that the following questions should be asked of a research report.

- Does the report attempt to link the problem with a theoretical framework?
- Is the theoretical framework tied to the study in a natural or contrived way?
- Would an alternative theoretical framework be more appropriate?
- Are the deductions from the theory logical?

In TFR researchers may not necessarily be generating theory nor may they be testing theoretical propositions in the form of hypotheses or research questions. Rather, the theory is used to frame the study and provide it with a focus. It could be argued that, so important is the theoretical framework, that researchers could more easily dispense with the physical operations of a study than the framework which gives meaning to all the research activity. The same methods could be used in a different study and give different outcomes if the conceptual framework were changed.

When used as a theoretical framework for a research report, theory:

- Gives direction to the investigation;
- Abstracts, summarises and orders research findings;
- Relates the study to previous work.

More specifically, Moody (1990) states that when a theory acts as a framework for research it serves to provide parameters for the study, guides in data collection and provides a perspective for interpreting the data so that the researcher is able to weave together the facts in a meaningful pattern. When a study is placed within a theoretical context, the theory guides the research process

from the research questions through design, analysis and interpretation to the conclusions. Silva (1986a) states that it is the
responsibility of the researcher to identify the theoretical framework for the study, however tentative it may seem in the beginning.
Linking the theory to the research guides the conduct of the study.

Batey (1971) asserts that, to be a source of knowledge, each
research study must be structured within a theoretical framework.
She maintains that the theoretical framework is the researcher's
organising image of the phenomena to be studied. Within TFR
the researcher's way of selecting certain things and searching for
patterns among them is guided by some prior notion or theories
about the nature of the phenomena under study. It is this theoretical framework which determines what questions will be addressed
by the study and how the data will be collected.

However, I have noted problems with TFR. It is possible that
researchers may include a theory into the beginning of a study to
lend the research report some theoretical credibility. In many
instances, the theory is not referred to again and it was, in reality,
merely 'window dressing'. A potentially more serious problem
relates to the inappropriate selection of a theory to frame the study.
As with selecting a theory for practice (see Chapter 5), such a
choice may lead to premature commitment to a particular theory
with the result that theoretical and clinical vision is restricted and a
clear understanding of the phenomena is blocked. For instance, a
social anthropological theory about family support developed in
New Guinea may not be appropriate when applied to nursing in the
UK. Similarly, a theory that focuses on self-care may ignore
patients who genuinely want the nurse to undertake all their care.

Therefore, the selection of a theoretical framework to underpin a
research study is a value-laden affair and influences:

● The problems deemed worthy of study;
● The perceived social benefits;
● The definitions and measurements of concepts;
● The types of participant risk worth taking;
● The acceptable threats to internal and external validity;
● The interpretation and significance of the findings;
● How the knowledge is used.

Therefore, a theoretical framework used to structure a research study may take on an agenda-setting role bringing with it inherent biases. As Reed (1989) puts it, the conceptual nets cast out by researchers could be used to catch fish only of their liking.

Ellis (1970) stressed that, unlike some scientists, the nurse researcher should ask 'why' when she starts a search for knowledge, and the answer should contain a relevance to nursing. Therefore, it is recommended that, in research that pertains to nursing practice, the theory framing the study should be a nursing one. Donaldson and Crowley (1978) differentiate between 'substantive structure' and 'syntactic structure'. The former refers to the scope and nature of enquiry in nursing, the latter refers to the methods and approaches of enquiry. The findings from the latter add to the former. When the relationship of nursing theory to the former is explicit, this leads the way to good research. They state that

> for the continued growth, significance and utility of a discipline of nursing, researchers must place their research within the context of the discipline. Theories must also be viewed in terms of the basic structural conceptualisations of the discipline. The responsibility for revising and clarifying the structural conceptions, the very framework of the discipline of nursing, rests with nurse researchers. This means lessening our preoccupation with the process of nursing and pedagogy and placing emphasis on content as substance.
>
> (Donaldson and Crowley, 1978: 120)

The substantive nature of a discipline will help determine the 'syntax'. For example, if we believe that what is of substantive importance for nursing is the patients' lived experiences then a phenomenological approach will be the obvious choice. If we maintain that unitary human beings are our focus, then our syntactic approaches will be concerned with looking for patterns with these beings. If physiological functioning is our substantive area, then a positivist approach will be appropriate (Salsberry, 1994). The lesson here is that if we mix and match methods without taking cognisance of the underlying substantive philosophy this will lead to confusion and a dilution of meaning (Smith, 1994).

In TFR, the findings may:

- Contribute indirectly to establishing the worth of the theory as a template for the study;
- Contribute indirectly to the generation of a new theory (Hunink, 1995);
- Lead to a rejection of an existing theory as a guide for a research study;
- Lead to an existing theory being adapted or revised.

Theory-evaluating research (TER)

While this may seem to be related to TTR, there are substantial differences. There is a body of opinion in the literature suggesting that grand theories cannot be tested and therefore the best we can do is evaluate their application in practice and education to see if they have any noticeable effect. Holden (1990) points out that while it may not be possible to test scientifically the underlying assumptions and propositions of some nursing theories it is possible to scrutinise certain aspects of nursing care affected by their introduction.

Acknowledging the lack of research on the effects of nursing theories, Chinn and Jacobs (1987) in the US and Walsh (1989) in the UK call for investigations to be carried out to determine the results of applying nursing theories. I would refer the reader to Chapter 6, where an overview is presented of research studies that focused on the effects of nursing theories in practice. For the remainder of this section I will present a brief summary of the TER within nurse education.

Despite the fact that nursing theories have been taught in the US and the UK for some years now, the amount of empirical research concerning their effect on nurse learning is conspicuous by its scarcity. In a recent British text on nursing theories Fraser (1996: 3) admitted that for many theories in nursing there is not a great deal of research available to date. Therefore, one must look to the United States for most of the investigations in this field.

Two American nurse educators, Hagemeier and Hunt (1979), constructed a thirteen-item Likert-type questionnaire to find out if

they had achieved their teaching objectives as far as nursing theories were concerned. They also wished to know if past graduates
were using nursing theories in their practice. Of 150 questionnaires
distributed, 69 were completed and returned. Results showed that
53 had a positive view of nursing theories, 5 had a negative view
and 11 were undecided in their response.

The majority of respondents had grasped the main teaching
objectives specified by the researchers. When asked if the nursing
theory provided them with a consistent approach in various nursing
situations, 63 per cent gave a positive response while 29 per cent
were undecided. The researchers conclude that the students' use of
a nursing theory during training positively influences their professional practice later on. However, the following methodological
issues must be recognised: the study was limited to sixty-nine
respondents from the same school of nursing, the questionnaire
was limited to thirteen items and no account is given of its reliability or validity.

Jacobson (1987) carried out a survey in the US to describe when
and how nurses acquire their knowledge of nursing theories and
how they regard them. The research subjects, graduate nursing students and their teachers, were presented with a forty-three item
questionnaire. Responses were obtained from 480 master's students,
112 doctoral students and 99 faculty members. Findings indicated
that 78 (12 per cent) were familiar with one theory, 128 (19 per
cent) with two, 247 (36 per cent) with three/four and 223 (33 per
cent) with five or more. When asked which theory they were familiar with, 259 said Orem, 244 Rogers, 217 Roy, 102 King, 102
Neuman, 56 Johnson, 37 Peplau, 35 Levine and twenty other theories received between one and eighteen responses each.

When asked about the use of nursing theories in the delivery of
care, only 244 (35 per cent) said that they had actually used a theory in practice. Most of the respondents (76 per cent) were
enthusiastic about nursing theories, with a statistically significant
difference among the three groups regarding this issue; 28 per cent
of the master's students and 23 per cent of the doctoral students
were uncertain or unenthusiastic; teachers were most enthusiastic
(88 per cent). When asked how important nursing theories were for
the advancement of nursing, 84 per cent of master's students, 96

per cent of doctoral students and 91 per cent of nurse teachers believed them to be 'crucial'.

Jacobson's study is one of the largest undertaken into the utilisation of and opinions on nursing theories. In the main, it appears to be well planned and executed. However, bias in the selection of potential respondents may have occurred due to the fact that 'contact persons' in the target schools were relied upon to supply the names of eligible subjects. Furthermore, only 54 per cent of all master's programmes and 32 per cent of all doctoral programmes were surveyed. Therefore, one cannot generalise the findings to all such programmes.

Jukes (1988) surveyed senior tutors and senior nurses in ten English health authorities concerning the frameworks used for assessment in the field of mental handicap. Using a postal questionnaire, he found that the majority used psychologically based assessment tools. Theories of nursing were mostly unacknowledged or unused in those areas where there were no strong links between education and service. With the exception of three health authorities, Jukes found that the introduction of nursing theories was mostly a 'classroom activity' (1988: 10).

Roper *et al.*'s theory was favoured by four out of the ten health authorities, Henderson's by two, Peplau's by one, Orem's by one and Roy's by one. Although exact figures are not given by Jukes, he does say that some see nursing theories as useful assessment tools whereas others do not. Jukes does not mention if the questionnaire was piloted or tested for reliability or validity; neither does he discuss how the respondents were selected. One must also question if senior tutors would necessarily be *au fait* with current assessment strategies at patient care level.

In 1991, Salanders and Dietz-Omar reported the results of an American survey into whether nurses believed nursing theories helped them in clinical decision making. Data were collected at three points in time: prior to taking a nursing theory course, on completion of the course, and two years later. At the first data collection point respondents were neutral in their responses, neither agreeing nor disagreeing when asked if nursing theories provided a frame of reference for their practice. However, at the two latter data collection points the respondents believed that nursing theories did indeed provide a frame of reference for clinical decision making.

Although Salanders and Dietz-Omar (1991) give detailed statistical results of their research, they omit to include all aspects relevant to methodology. Without this information one cannot judge the relevance or otherwise of these findings.

As with theory evaluation in nursing practice (see Chapter 6), a review of the literature on TER in nurse education demonstrates that published investigations are relatively few in number. Most reports tend to concentrate on findings rather than method. This leaves the reader at a disadvantage if replication or generalisation is desired.

In TER, the findings may:

- Contribute to establishing the worth of the theory in practice or education;
- Contribute to the generation of ideas for new theory;
- Lead to a rejection of an existing theory as a guide for practice or curricula;
- Lead to an existing theory being adapted or revised within practice or education.

Theory and research – the view of metatheorists

Dickoff and James's (1968) four levels of theory have been discussed in previous chapters. In Table 7.1 their relationship with research methods is illustrated.

Building on Dickoff and James's (1968) view of a hierarchy of theories, it is possible to identify three main types of theory and their related research methods:

Descriptive theory: there are two types of descriptive theory – naming theories and taxonomies (classification theories). Descriptive theories are generated and tested by descriptive research generally called descriptive/exploratory research. The sorts of research questions asked within descriptive studies are: What is this? What are the characteristics of . . .? Descriptive studies involve the observation of phenomena in their natural setting. Data collection can be qualitative (e.g., case studies, ethnography, phenomenology, grounded

Table 7.1 The relationship between levels of theory and levels of research

Dickoff and James (1968)	Diers (1979)
Factor-isolating theory: describes and names concepts.	Factor-naming or factor-searching research: describes, names a phenomenon, situation or event in order to gain new insights – called descriptive or exploratory research.
Factor-relating theory relates named concepts to one another.	Factor-relating/relation or factor-searching research: develops links among variables and describes the relationships that are discovered after factor-searching research – may be qualitative or grounded theory.
Situation-relating theories: interrelationship between concepts or propositions.	Explanatory/correlational research: aims to determine factors that occur or vary together – no attempt is made to experiment.
Situation-producing theory: prescribes actions to reach certain outcomes.	Causal-hypothesis testing: research addresses causal relationships between variables in an attempt to predict events.

theory, etc.) or quantitative (surveys of attitudes, attributes, knowledge and opinions).

Explanatory theory: this type of theory specifies relations between dimensions or characteristics of individuals, groups, situations or events. It sets out to explain how the parts of the phenomena under study relate to each other. These theories can only be formulated once phenomena have been identified through descriptive theories having previously been developed. Explanatory theories are developed through explanatory (qualitative) or correlational (quantitative) studies. An example of a research question would be: To what extent is age related to dependency?

Data for explanatory theories may be collected through the use of surveys (observations, interviews, questionnaires) yielding quantitative or qualitative data; fixed-choice tools may be used because the parts of the phenomena are believed to be already known as a result of the existence of descriptive theories. To prove a correlation, qualitative data may be transformed into quantitative data and statistical tests such as Pearson Product Moment Co-efficient (parametric) or Spearman's Rho (non-parametric) used. Other more sophisticated tests such as multiple regression or path analysis may also be used.

Predictive theory: this type of theory goes beyond whether one thing is related to another and seeks to identify cause and effect relationships. Predictive theories may build on explanatory theories and are generated and tested by experimental research. Questions addressed include: What will happen if you give specific information before surgery? Quantitative data are required to seek statistical significance. Tests include Mann-Whitney U-test (non-parametric) and T-test (parametric).

Therefore, if little is known about the phenomena, descriptive (descriptive theory) research is required. However, if phenomena have been adequately described, correlational (explanatory theory) research may be carried out. If phenomena have been adequately described and relationships are well known then experimental (predictive theory) research may be carried out (see Figure 7.4). Quantitative and qualitative methods are mutually supportive and can provide the researcher with binocular vision of the phenomena under study which neither can provide when used in isolation.

From Chapter 2 you will recall that Carper (1978) identified four different ways of knowing in nursing. Although they do not substantiate their claim to my satisfaction, Fawcett and Downs (1992) refer to these as theories. None the less, Chinn and Kramer (1995) demonstrate how each is guided by a particular mode of enquiry (see Box 7.2).

THEORY:	Descriptive	Explanatory	Predictive
	Qualitative	Qualitative	
RESEARCH:	Descriptive	Explanatory	Quantitative
	Quantitative Descriptive	Quantitative Correlational	Experimental

Figure 7.4 The relationship between types of theory and research methods

---

Box 7.2 Chinn and Kramer's ways of knowing and modes of enquiry

Way of knowing	*Mode of enquiry*
Empirics:	Scientific research
Ethics:	Dialogue about justice
Personal knowing:	Reflection on the congruity between the authentic and disclosed selves
Aesthetics:	Critique of the act of nursing

Strategies for theory development through research

Meleis (1991) identifies five major strategies for theory development:

- Theory–practice–theory
- Practice–theory
- Research–theory
- Theory–research–theory
- Practice–theory–research–theory.

Theory–practice–theory strategy

Here, theory from other disciplines is implemented in nursing and becomes shared knowledge. For example, the application from psychology of interpersonal theory in psychiatric nursing practice led to the formulation of Peplau's (1952) theory. Similarly, existentialist theory when applied in psychiatry led to the development of Travelbee's (1966) theory.

Practice–theory strategy

The discerning reader will note the relationship of this strategy to TGR. According to Meleis, here theory emanates from clinical experience and there may or may not be an existing theory which guides the theorist in how he or she views the phenomena. The process usually starts when the clinician has a nagging hunch about some phenomena. He or she develops concepts and describes definitions, boundaries and examples of these concepts. This strategy is heavily based upon Glaser and Strauss's (1967) grounded theory approach where the theorist keeps diaries, observes, analyses similarities and differences, develops concepts and then linkages. Orlando (1961), Wiedenbach (1964) and Travelbee (1966) used these methods, becoming totally immersed in the clinical area, either giving care themselves or observing others giving care. They collected data using case studies, interviews and observations.

Research–theory strategy

This strategy is also related to TGR. This is an inductive approach using four steps:

1 Select a phenomenon that occurs frequently – list all its characteristics;
2 Measure characteristics in a variety of settings;
3 Analyse resultant data to determine systematic patterns worthy of further attention;
4 Formalise these patterns as theoretical statements (axioms).

(Reynolds 1971: 140)

Proponents of this strategy believe truth exists that can be captured through the senses and verified or falsified. Repeated verification is indicative of truth and prompts the development of scientific theories. Not all supporters of this strategy advocate sensory data and verification or falsification as a basis of truth. Grounded theorists also use this strategy for the discovery of concepts, identification of patterns and explanations.

Theory–research–theory strategy

This strategy shows similarities with the TTR approaches outlined above. The following four steps are followed:

1 A theory is selected that explains the phenomena of interest;
2 Concepts of the theory are redefined and operationalised for research;
3 Findings are synthesised and used to modify, refine or develop the original theory;
4 In some instances the result may be a new theory.

Practice–theory–research–theory strategy

There are seven stages in this strategy and readers may note similarities with Walker and Avant's (1995) concept analysis process as outlined in Chapter 3. The stages are:

1 taking in
2 description of phenomenon
3 labelling
4 concept development
5 propositional development
6 explicating assumptions
7 sharing and communicating.

Meleis (1991) states that these seven steps may not occur linearly; rather, they may occur simultaneously or out of sequence.

1 *Taking in*: a clinical situation has attracted your attention and you develop a hunch about it. You may have observed this event not only through your eyes but through your senses and

through mental activity. The result is 'attention grabbing' which may occur concurrently or retrospectively. The *attention grabbing* phase is followed by the *attention giving* phase, a more deliberate process. You may ask the following questions:

- What has attracted my attention?
- Why does it happen?
- Is it similar to or different from happenings under different sets of circumstances?
- Under what conditions do I observe it, see it, hear it, touch it?
- Can I describe it?
- Can I document it with theory cases and prototype situations?

2 *Description of phenomenon*: at this second stage you should attempt to answer a further set of questions:

- What is the phenomenon?
- When does it occur?
- What are its boundaries?
- Does it vary? Under what circumstances?
- Does it have a function?
- Is it related to time or place?

Another way to begin the description of a phenomenon is by asking questions which start:

- Why do patients . . .?
- What is it that happens when . . .?
- What are the properties of...?

To ensure that the phenomena are of specific interest to nurses and nursing it is a good idea to attempt answers to the following questions:

- In what way is the phenomenon related to nursing's substantive knowledge base?
- In what way would understanding the phenomenon contribute to understanding some aspect of nursing care?
- Can I think of some questions relating to the phenomenon, the answers to which would be significant to nursing?
- How is the phenomenon related to what nursing policy is?

For instance, a nurse may observe how children cry inconsolably as visiting time ends yet stop immediately once their parents have left the ward. This is a beginning observation that may evolve into a phenomenon. As similar observations occur the nurse can ask questions of other staff, read and reflect. The end result would be an in-depth description of a phenomenon.

3 *Labelling*: in the paediatric case the nurse labels the phenomenon with a word or a short phrase. What she is in essence doing is identifying a concept which best reflects the phenomenon. From Chapter 3 you will remember that these labels should be concise and precise, used consistently when referring to the phenomenon, contain one cardinal idea and be fundamental to the definition/description of the phenomenon. In the above case, the nurse may label the observed phenomenon 'temporary separation distress'.

4 *Concept development*: the following techniques have been identified by Meleis (1991) as appropriate ways of developing new concepts:
- *Defining*: here you seek definitions/synonyms of the concept.
- *Differentiating*: here you ask: How does this concept differ from similar concepts?
- *Delineating antecedents*: here you define the context and part of this relates to identifying what precedes the occurrence of the concept.
- *Delineating consequences*: here you identify what results from, or follows, the occurrence of the concept. Positive as well as negative consequences should be identified.
- *Modelling*: here both contrary and like cases are identified to help depict what the concept is and what it is not.
- *Analogising*: here the concept is compared to similar concepts which have been studied more extensively. This may help to shed more light on what the new concept is.
- *Synthesising*: here you bring together the findings, meanings and properties that have been amplified by the previous processes.

5   *Propositional development*: propositions may be developed to describe the properties of the concept. This development of propositional statements is a further step in the process of theory development. As outlined above, there are different types of proposition and the more developed propositions are, the more they are able to define, explain and predict the nature of the relationship between concepts.

6   *Explicating assumptions*: the observer reflects on the concepts and propositions and identifies both explicit and implicit assumptions. Reflections on one's own views, values and beliefs will help to delineate assumptions.

7   *Sharing and communicating*: this step goes beyond publishing and presenting at conferences. It involves seminars, conference presentations, journal clubs and other forums where theoretical issues are discussed.

In conclusion, it is important that nurse researchers are acutely aware of the part their study will play in the development or testing of theory. One way of checking this is to answer the following questions:

- What is the nature and scope of the research aims: exploratory, descriptive, explanatory, predictive?
- Did an existing theory provide the initial idea for the research?
- Is the aim of the study to test existing concepts or propositions from a theory?
- Were study concepts or propositions derived from an existing theory?
- Is the purpose of the study to describe or understand phenomena and from these phenomena develop descriptive or explanatory theory?
- What predominant world view is reflected in the nature of the research questions (e.g., totality versus simultaneity)?
- Has there been much theoretical progress undertaken on this particular topic?

(Moody, 1990)

Summary

There are three core elements in any practice discipline. These are research, theory and practice. This chapter has attempted to identify a range of relationships between all three. However, particular emphasis was paid to the linkages between research and theory. Four links were identified: theory-testing research, theory-generating research, theory-framed research and theory-evaluating research. All four were discussed at length and their contribution to the knowledge base of nursing was explored.

Various metatheorists have also examined the linkages between theory, practice and research. Meleis, for instance, identified five distinct strategies highlighting the linkages. Chinn and Kramer built on Carper's work and specified how the four ways of knowing are related to methods of enquiry. Similarly, Donna Diers constructed a taxonomy of research–theory relationships by building on the work of Dickoff and James.

Oliver Slevin (1996) asks us to imagine that theory, practice and research are three dancers. This is a useful metaphor. The dancers interact to produce a systematic and aesthetic beauty and elegance. One weak dancer who stumbles or does not undertake the appropriate movements would cause problems for all three, and such a passenger can only be 'carried' for so long. Therefore, all three partners need to be strong and skilled. Similarly, research with weak theory or practice with weak research would be the death-knell of nursing as a discipline. It is in our interests to keep these three components strong and ensure that they interact appropriately.

Chapter 8
Analysis and critique of nursing theory

Any approach constructed to describe, analyse and evaluate nursing theories must be systematic and rigorous. Since the mid-1960s numerous attempts have been made to present the perfect scheme. All have their limitations, because invariably some sort of judgement is called for. This can be due to the inherent biases of the developer or the user of the scheme. Considering that most nursing theories are abstract, it is not surprising that a structured list of criteria is often inadequate to judge their worth. Furthermore, since many nursing theories have their roots in an interpretative/historicist philosophy (see Chapter 2), it seems contradictory to evaluate these theories using rigid empiricist principles and rules.

A theory should not be accepted unquestioningly. Describing a theory is really about providing facts about it. This is useful in that it outlines the structure of the theory, its concepts, propositions and assumptions. Theory analysis goes a stage further; it is a systematic process of examining if the theory is valid in its composition and function. According to Moody (1990), the purpose of theory analysis is to identify the theory's degree of usefulness as a device to guide practice, education and administration and in its potential to influence the development of testable hypotheses and researchable questions. A further stage is theory evaluation or critique. Here, the theory's contribution to the development of scientific knowledge is assessed. Moody (1990) states that evaluation is about judging the worth of the theory.

Metatheorists in nursing have deliberated a great deal on what criteria should be used to analyse and evaluate theories. Some who take a pragmatist view believe that theories are only useful if they make a positive difference to practice; but others accept that many grand theories are almost too abstract for practice and their worth lies in making practitioners think about their discipline in creative and interesting ways. There are others who want the best of both worlds and are happiest with a pluralist repertoire of grand, mid-range and practice theories. Therefore, the description, analysis and evaluation of a theory is not a straightforward enterprise and should not be taken lightly.

The theoretical literature abounds with frameworks drawn up for this purpose. In essence, most are made up of features and topics that all theories have in common. These features are condensed within a scheme that forms a means of comparing numerous theories and their respective emphases. The following metatheorists have published such schemes: Dickoff and James (1968), Riehl and Roy (1980), Meleis (1991), Stevens-Barnum (1994), Chinn and Kramer (1995), Fawcett (1995), Walker and Avant (1995), and Fitzpatrick and Whall (1996). Controversy exists among many of these authors as to which scheme is the best. This contributes to the confusion that already exists at practitioner level. However, a review of these schemes reveals similarities. For instance, almost all are constructed around the metaparadigm of 'person', 'health', 'nursing' and the 'environment'. This is hardly surprising, considering that these elements form the mainframe of all theories in nursing and each theory is merely a representation of how the particular theorist views these elements.

Below, an attempt is made to extract the best criteria from a range of existing evaluative and analytical schemes. You will note that the criteria identified as meaningful have much in common with those identified as being helpful for theory selection (see Chapter 5).

The following categories could be usefully incorporated in an appropriate analytic and evaluative scheme.

- How the theory was developed;
- How the theory is internally structured;
- How the theory may be used;
- How the theory influences knowledge development;
- How the theory stands up to testing.

How the theory was developed

When analysing a theory you should take cognisance of its philosophical and geographic origins (Fawcett, 1995). This may include an exploration of the theorist's background, both educationally and experientially. For instance, would a theorist whose background was surgical nursing be credible as an originator of a mental health nursing theory? You may also wish to explore the motivation for developing the theory: was it developed as part of a doctoral thesis, as course work for a master's assignment or to structure care in a particular facility? Roy (1971) recalls how her theory was stimulated by a challenge from her teacher, Dorothy Johnson. Betty Neuman's (1995) theory was developed almost by accident when her early work was confused with that of the established theorist, Margaret Newman (1979).

Information about the theorist can be found in the primary sources of the literature, and several metatheorists, for example Marriner-Tomey (1994) and Fitzpatrick and Whall (1996), provide biographies of most of the major theorists. Interestingly, according to Peplau (1987), most of the nurse theorists are unmarried, childless and female. Hunink (1995) suggests that this is because there are fewer male nurses in the United States compared to Europe. This fact may also be important when reflecting on how the work of these theorists has been considered in a male-dominated health care and scientific world.

From Chapter 2 you may recall that, philosophically, two main methods for the development of theory have been identified: the inductive approach and the deductive approach. The inductive method leads to the development of theory based upon evidence drawn from observation and personal experience. In this case, the 'theorist' is reasoning from the 'specific' to the 'general' (the research-then-theory approach). In contrast, the deductive method leads to the development of theory from existing theories where reasoning is from the 'general' to the 'specific' (theory-then-research approach).

Although some theorists maintain that they derived their theories inductively from observing and working in practice (Roy, 1971; Orem, 1980), most take as their starting-point other theories.

For instance, Roy (1971) based her idea of adaptation on Harry Helson's theory of how the rods and cones of the eye adapt to light. Peplau (1952) was strongly influenced by the interpersonal theory propounded by Henry Stack Sullivan. Roper, Logan and Tierney's (1990) work demonstrates a clear link to that of Henderson's (1966) theory, and Henderson's work was based on Abraham Maslow's (1954) motivational theory. More recently, the origins of Parse's (1981) work and Fitzpatrick's (1982) work can be traced to the influence of Martha Roger's (1970) theory. Theories have also been deduced from the broad paradigms discussed in Chapter 4. These are the systems paradigm, the interactional paradigm, the developmental paradigm and the behavioural paradigm.

However, while many of the theories that currently exist in nursing have been deduced from other theories or paradigms, there is evidence that clinical practice also influenced their development. Therefore, when undertaking an analysis, you should establish whether a mixture of induction and deduction (i.e. retroduction) was used in the development of a theory. For example, while a mid-range theory on caring may have been developed inductively using a 'grounded theory' approach, it may have been tested deductively in other settings.

You should also consider the influence of socio-cultural factors. For instance, in the mid- to late 1960s 'flower power', freedom and the respect of others became a social movement. Such humanist influences can be detected in the work of Travelbee (1966) and Hall (1966). The political and cultural time frame for development is also of interest. Early theorists were interested in *what* nursing was and *what* nurses did, later theorists were interested in *how* nurses did what they did and, more recently, theorists are interested in *why* nurses do what they do.

This indicates that nursing theories are in a continual state of flux. Feedback from research, from practising nurses, from students and from colleagues provides theorists with a wealth of suggestions for altering and strengthening their work. Callista Roy (1996), for example, has changed some of the terminology relating to the 'four adaptation modes' within her theory, and shortly before her death Martha Rogers changed her theory's central concept of 'four-dimensionally' to 'pan-dimensionally'. Orem is another theorist whose work has not stagnated. She publishes a new edition of her book every five years. It is a useful exercise to look back at theorists' early publications and see how their work has changed and how theoretical status has been strengthened. Theorists who, in the 1950s to 1970s, referred to their work as conceptual models began calling them theories in the 1980s and 1990s.

It is also an interesting exercise to try to determine what philosophy of science is favoured by different theorists. Henderson's (1966) and Roper, Logan and Tierney's (1990) work seem to reflect an empiricist philosophy while Parse (1981) used an interpretative/historicist philosophy. You should also consider if the theory was based upon a rationalist philosophy whereby the theorist generated her ideas by reasoning. For instance, Orem (1980) remembers when she got the idea for her theory on self-care. She described how it came to her as an 'aha' experience. You should also consider whether a well-established theory will still be as valid and viable in the twenty-first century. As alluded to elsewhere, the simultaneity theories (see Chapter 4) may gain increased recognition and the totality theories may be redundant other than for archival purposes.

How the theory is internally structured

The internal structure of theories is a core issue for analysis. The following criteria merit consideration.

Clarity

Perhaps one of the most important aspects of a theory is its clarity. Clarity may be rated as high or low. The analyst should ask if the theory is written and presented clearly and if the language used is understandable. This represents *semantic clarity*. You should ask the following questions: Are key terms defined? Are concepts and assumptions implicit? If explicit, are they stated clearly? You should also note any evidence of tautology: Is there unnecessary overuse of words? Note too if there is *structural clarity*. This occurs when the prepositional links between the concepts are clear to the reader and any diagram representing the theory can be understood without a great deal of difficulty. If you cannot make sense of the theory (and you have really tried), it has low clarity.

Simplicity

The theory should be elegant in its simplicity; that is, the theorist should have chosen the simplest, most parsimonious format possible to get across the theoretical message. If we want theory, practice and research to link appropriately, theory should be easily understood if it is to gain the attention and commitment of the hard-pressed clinicians. How can anyone use a theory if they cannot comprehend it? This applies equally well to diagrammatic representations. If a theory is composed of a confusing mixture of geometric lines, circles, triangles and squares, busy practitioners will not be impressed.

Considering the complexity of nursing, all theories cannot be presented in a simple manner. You may think a theory is complex and accept this fact because its concepts and assumptions relate to very difficult issues within practice. Therefore, you should make a judgement as to whether you think a theory is excessively simple or unnecessarily complicated in its content and form.

Consistency

All the components within the theory should support each other and be free from contradictions. As with clarity, consistency can be rated high or low. Look carefully to note if inconsistencies are explicit or implicit. Stevens-Barnum (1994) identified the following types of inconsistency:

- *Inconsistency in terms*: are definitions of concepts consistent with later assumptions? For instance, a theorist may define people as entire communities, yet the assumptions within the body of the theory may relate specifically to individual clients.
- *Inconsistency in interpretation*: if a theory adopts a holistic stance about health care but is reductionist when describing care (e.g., having a large biophysical emphasis).
- *Inconsistency in principle*: a theory may highlight the importance of clients being able to have choices yet be prescriptive in

the interventions it supports. Furthermore, inconsistency in principle may be observed when a theory that has its basis in a behavioural paradigm includes concepts that are better related to a system's paradigm.

- *Inconsistency in method*: a theory may have its origins in phenomenology or existentialism yet the theorist recommends empiricist approaches for its application and testing.

Metaparadigm

You should examine closely how the metaparadigm components are stated within the theory. What does the theorist have to say about the nature of people, the environment, health and nursing? Are these components and the assumptions relating to them made explicit? Does the theorist emphasise one to the detriment of others? For instance, while Florence Nightingale's (1859) and Martha Rogers's (1970) theories both deal with all metaparadigmatic elements, they concentrate their attention on the components 'people' and 'environment' and the relationship between them. You may also wish to check whether the relationships between the metaparadigm elements are stated clearly and if there is a transparent presentation or explanation of the beliefs and values and the goals associated with them.

If a theorist refers to 'persons', is she referring to patients, potential patients, communities or societies at large? When 'nursing' is mentioned is it the profession, the art, the science of nursing which is being alluded to, or the nursing act? Does 'environment' mean external environment or internal environment? Is 'health' a state of well-being, a physical status or a psycho-social feeling or indeed a state of becoming? It is important that you are clear as to what the theorist means when they refer either implicitly or explicitly to the metaparadigm.

Adequacy

A theory is adequate if it accounts for the subject-matter with which it deals (Stevens-Barnum, 1994). If a theory was specifically designed from experiences in acute psychiatric nursing in the

United Kingdom, and if the theorist claimed that its propositions could apply transculturally to all of nursing, this may well show up an inadequacy: the theory would probably not be transculturally applicable. I was privileged to teach nursing theory at the University of Malawi in southern Africa. The nurses there wanted to use the work Roy or Orem and other American theorists, believing them to be the 'gold standard'. They placed such theories on a pedestal and did not consider whether or not they were appropriate for their culture. It was better to enable them to design their own grand theory for Malawian nursing. When compared with American and British theories, this fledgling theory, and the concepts, propositions and assumptions within it, reflected at least the beginnings of adequacy.

Some theories, such as that of Peplau (1952), are adequate for mental health nursing but may prove to be inadequate when applied to acute surgical nursing. The same applies to Roy's theory (1996); it may be entirely adequate for acute surgical nursing but inadequate for care of the elderly.

Sound reasoning

Whether a theory was developed deductively or inductively, the reader must be sure that the reasoning processes were sound; in other words, that the theoretical conclusions are supportive of any preceding premises (see Chapter 2). You may ask whether the conclusions reached by the theory are legitimate when you take into account the premises; for instance, in a mid-range theory there may be the following reasoning:

- All patients are actively involved in decision making concerning their care (premise 1);
- People suffering from depression are patients (premise 2);
- Depressed patients are not involved in decision making (conclusion).

If the theory condoned such a conclusion then the reasoning is faulty.

Concepts and propositions

You should ask what position the concepts and propositions hold on the concrete-to-abstract continuum. Because concepts are the building blocks of theories you should check to ensure that they are clearly defined and that the way they have been joined together to form propositions seems acceptable. The following questions should be asked: Do the propositional statements seem valid, logical and relevant to the underlying philosophy of the theory? Have hypotheses been identified and if so are they testable or do they have empirical support? Have the concepts and propositions been presented in diagrammatic form?

Each theory has a set of propositions called assumptions or suppositions. From Chapter 1 you will recall that these are statements which we accept as true and take for granted. One of Roy's (1980) eight assumptions is that the person is a bio-psycho-social being. One of Orem's (1980) six assumptions is that self-care encourages positive self-esteem. Readers should carefully consider the assumptions of a theory and ask whether you can accept them as true.

How the theory is used

We are a practice profession and most of our theories should relate to practice. Accepting this, theories may also be useful as curricula guides within nursing education, may be the focus of investigation within research or form the philosophy for organisational management.

Dorothy Johnson (1959), in making an early attempt to specify by what means a theory should be analysed, centred on the theory's usefulness in practice and its value to the profession. She identified social utility, social significance and social congruence as useful criteria for analysis.

Social utility

Does the theory include explicit rules for practice? In other words, you should explore whether the theory suggests ways in which nurses should care for people. Under this category you should also look for evidence that the theory can help practitioners predict consequences from its use, prescribe actions which make a difference as well as describe and explain phenomena. You may wish to ask if the theory is concerned with practice as it is or as it ought to be.

Social significance

Does the theory lead to actions that make important differences for the client? This is a difficult question to answer, especially if the theory has not been tested. It relates to whether positive client outcomes are achieved through the use of interventions suggested by the theory. You could include under social significance the effect the theory has on quality of care. Although this includes outcomes, it also includes the interventions to be carried out and the resources needed to undertake best practice.

Social congruence/acceptance

Does the theory lead to activities that meet the expectations of society? You must examine whether the theory coincides with what society expects of nurses. For instance, if the theory encourages self-care, is it possible that in some cultures this would conflict with the pervading idea that the client is ill and therefore should accept a dependent role? Time and history are also important issues to consider under this category. A theory that was acceptable in the mid-nineteenth century (Nightingale, 1859) or mid-twentieth century (e.g. Peplau, 1952) may not be congruent with society's values and beliefs in the late 1990s.

It is important to note who perceives the theory to have social utility, significance and congruence. It may be that you cannot detect the presence of these factors in the theory, but many authors and metatheorists in the literature state that they are present. Do not be afraid to be true to your own feelings, as long as you can explain your reasons for disagreeing with others. Sometimes it is good to veer from compliance with the opinion of others and state your own opinions.

Scope/generality

This relates to how the theory can be applied and its degree of abstractness. You can rate the scope/generality of the theory on a continuum between broad and narrow. The theory may be a grand theory providing a broad philosophical abstraction of the reality of nursing. Alternatively, it may be a mid-theory which has been based upon research findings and is easily applicable to a specific group of patients. Perhaps it is a practice theory offering clinically oriented explicit guides for nursing actions so that desired outcomes can be achieved.

A grand theory such as Orem's self-care theory (1980) may be used in a variety of different cultures because all people have self-care needs and some require nursing care when they are incapable of undertaking self-care. Other theories may be narrower in their scope and their generalisability is limited. An example of this would be Wewers and Lenz's (1987) theory of relapse among ex-smokers.

However, in some cases the generalisability of a theory may not be related to its scope. For instance, one grand theory may be applicable world-wide while another may be only suitable to Western countries. It is also possible that a practice theory could have a broad scope. For example, the practice theory relating to two-hourly turning for pressure sore prevention may be applicable throughout the world. The same may apply to the practice theory of pre-operative information-giving having a positive outcome in terms of post-operative recovery. This relatively narrow-range theory may be as applicable in New Guinea as it is in the UK.

It could be argued that the broader the scope of a theory, the greater the possibility that it will be more 'socially congruent' (see above). As Hardy (1991) asserts, a theory of grieving that can be applied to all ages and cultures is more useful than a theory of grieving that relates only to middle-aged individuals in the US who have lost their spouse. In contrast, the narrower the scope of a theory the higher its 'social utility'. Furthermore, since broad theories are not easily testable, there is the possibility that they would have low 'social significance'.

Guidance for the nursing process

All theories influence aspects of the decision-making and problem-solving strategy that is the nursing process. In particular, each
grand theory describes its version of the 'process', frequently in
great detail. Some theories identify a four-stage (Roper, Logan and
Tierney, 1990), a five-stage (Orem, 1985) or a six-stage 'process'
(Roy, 1971).

Therefore, a nursing theory should bring the nursing process to
life. It specifies what should be assessed, what interventions to use
and how care can be evaluated. The 'process' is an empty procedure
without a theory to structure it. By providing this guidance, the theory is, either explicitly or implicitly, specifying the role of the nurse
in the delivery of health care, indicating as it does the focus and
mode of intervention. You should be aware that some nursing theories can be good templates for assessment but may not offer
explicit guidance for action or evaluation.

Accessibility

Chinn and Kramer (1995) include accessibility as an important criterion for analysis. This relates to whether the theory has empirical
indicators that reflect its concepts. If not, it would be difficult to
test the theory in the real world of practice. Most grand theories
have not got explicit empirical indicators; in contrast, most mid-
range and practice theories have.

Reality convergence

This concept relates to whether the theory's view of the world con-
forms to that of the potential user (Stevens-Barnum, 1994).
Suppose you firmly believe that there are three dimensions to our
existence: height, width and depth. Your views of reality would
not converge with that of Rogers (1980), who argues that there are
four dimensions (now pan-dimension) to our existence. You would
have difficulty using this theory to guide your thinking and practice
if your views were at odds with those of the theorist. This does not
mean it is a bad theory, only that its perspective, assumptions and
beliefs do not coincide with your own.

As part of your deliberations you should also reflect on whether or not you like this theory, and why. Practising nurses may be attracted to a particular theory without really knowing the reason. Perhaps it does converge with their beliefs and values or perhaps it is understandable or easily applied in practice. Alternatively, for equally uncertain reasons, a nurse may reject what would appear to be a suitable theory. Sometimes nurses, especially expert nurses, have to 'follow their heart' when it comes to a theory. If, later, they find that the theory was not appropriate for their needs, they can move to another.

Discrimination

Nursing is a discrete discipline whose view of phenomena may differ in perspective compared to that of other disciplines. You should seek to find out if the theory has the capacity to differentiate those who provide nursing from other health professionals and from informal family carers (Stevens-Barnum, 1994). This is an essential quality in any applied profession that borrows many of its scientific ideas from other disciplines. If a nursing theory does not show how nursing is unique compared to other disciplines, then one would wonder if it was a nursing theory at all. It would be a good exercise to remove the word 'nursing' from Orem's self-care theory (1980) or Henderson's (1966) activities of living theory and present them to occupational therapists or physiotherapists. If, upon studying them, these disciplines believed that the theories were suitable for their practice, then concern about the theories' discrimination should be expressed.

Circle of contagiousness

In the United Kingdom we have imported several American theories. Meleis (1991) would refer to this geographical spread of a theory, not directly influenced by the theorist, as the 'widening circle of contagiousness'. In your analysis, you may wish to note whether the theory has been altered in its transcultural, cross-frontier journey and who was directly responsible for its introduction in this country. You may also wish to ask: Within what specialty is it being used? How is it being used? Is it used to structure practice, curricula and/or research? Is the theory being used by other health professionals, such as occupational therapists or social workers? If so, in what way?

How the theory influences knowledge development

Theory generation

When analysing a theory you should explore whether the theory has the potential to generate other theories. For example, Rogers (1980) influenced the development of Fitzpatrick's (1982) theory. A grand theory may suggest new avenues of exploration, which can lead to the development of mid-range and practice theories. You may also want to discover if the resultant theories will be descriptive, explanatory, predictive or prescriptive (see Chapter 7).

Importance

This concerns whether the theory is forward-looking and whether it is a valuable resource in the creation of a desired future (Chinn and Kramer, 1995). This desired future may be related to the advancement of practice, the underpinning of research studies or as a framework for curricular development in education. With 'importance', you are examining whether in your opinion, and in that of others (colleagues or literature sources), the theory will help or hinder the development of your discipline. Take the former: as a consequence of using it, the theory may have the potential to answer questions or resolve problems that are central to nursing's future. Supporting this, Hardy (1991) asks us to consider whether the theory gives a sense of insight or suggests new ideas or new ways of looking at phenomena.

How the theory stands up to testing

Theory testing

You will recall from Chapter 7 that a major reason for the existence of theories is to guide and be guided by research. Propositions within theories can be developed into testable hypotheses and these in turn can be subjected to investigation which can result in the development of new knowledge. You may find in most cases that many of these theories have not been tested by researchers, the theorists themselves or by those nurses who use them in practice.

There has been a great deal written about the necessity of testing theories to provide evidence of the validity and accuracy of their concepts and assumptions (Chinn and Jacobs, 1987). However, little progress has been made towards this goal. Dickoff and James (1968) recommend such testing, claiming that not to do so would have consequences for the quality of care. This is understandable considering the implications of nurses and midwives using a theory of dubious validity as an organising framework for the care of clients.

Following a comprehensive search of the American literature from 1952 to 1985, Mary Silva (1986b) found that the use of research to test the assumptions of theories was rare. She said that this was an aspect of science that had remained outside the nursing research mainstream.

Silva used the following rigid selection criteria:

- The research is to determine the validity of a theory's assumptions/prepositions;
- The theory is an explicit framework for the research;
- The relationship between the theory and the study's hypotheses is clear;
- The research hypotheses are deduced clearly from the theory's assumptions;
- The research hypotheses are tested in an appropriate manner;
- The research provides indirect evidence as to the validity of the theory's assumptions/prepositions;
- The evidence is discussed in terms of how it supports, refutes or explains the theory.

Concentrating on the work of one or more of five theorists – Roy, Orem, Newman, Rogers and Johnson – Silva located sixty-two research studies which seemed to be testing theory. She categorised them into three groups:

1 *Minimal use*: in these studies the theory was used as a framework for the research but was not integrated further into the study. Of the sixty-two studies twenty-four were in this category.
2 *Insufficient use*: in these studies the theory was only used to organise the research instruments. Of the sixty-two studies twenty-nine were in this category.
3 *Adequate use*: in these studies the researchers met the seven criteria outlined above. However, of the sixty-two studies Silva identified only nine in this category, several of which she felt tested only a part of the theory.

Silva concluded that many studies have used theories as frameworks for research but only a few have explicitly tested these theories in the sense of trying to determine the underlying validity of the model's assumptions or propositions (1986b: 8).

Two years later, Moody *et al.* (1988) analysed 720 research articles published in six of the major nursing research journals focusing on nursing practice research. She wanted to see how many of the studies attempted to test nursing theory. She found that there was a link between the research design and a theory in 55 per cent of the studies (half were at descriptive level of theory). Less than thirty-five had tested the concepts or hypotheses of a theory. The most frequently used theory in the studies analysed was Orem, followed by Rogers, Newman and Roy. Surprisingly, 89 per cent of the research articles reviewed reported no nursing theory. None the less, Moody calculated that between 1977 and 1986 there was a statistically significant increase in nursing theories being used for research purposes. In 1977, 52 per cent of the studies used a theory from another discipline compared with 49 per cent in 1986. The three most frequently cited non-nursing theories were Lazarus's theory of coping (twenty-seven studies), the health belief model of Becker and Rosenstock (twenty-five studies) and the locus of control from social learning theory (twelve studies).

Therefore, of the 720 research studies examined by Moody *et al.* (1988) 10 per cent reported some level of usage of a nursing theory and only 3 per cent actually set out to test concepts or hypotheses from nursing theories. Other American 'theory watchers' who have undertaken similar literature searches to that of Silva have come up with comparable findings. In reviewing the journal *Nursing Research* for the years 1974 to 1985, Beck (1985) noted that only a 'few' research studies involved the testing of nursing theories. In 1989 Allen and Hayes undertook a similar project. They found that little had changed in the four years since Silva's work.

However, as alluded to elsewhere, there is a section of the literature which argues that because of their conceptual make-up grand theories cannot be tested. For example, Kristjanson, Tamblyn and Kuypers (1987) maintain that such theories do not provide the level of specificity required to derive and test principles. Fawcett (1990) asserts that because the propositions of a grand theory are so abstract and general, and because the concepts are not operationally defined, they are not amenable to testing. There is also the belief that, since many theories are more philosophic than scientific, the lack of empirical testing is justified (Uys, 1987). Therefore, you might like to consider as part of your analysis whether untested theories should be used to underpin client care.

Summary

Clients deserve care which, theoretically and practically, is the best that can be given. Therefore, an important part of knowledge development is the analysis of theories. In this chapter I have described how you may approach this by working through five evaluative categories:

- How the theory was developed;
- How the theory is structured;
- How the theory may be used;
- How the theory influences knowledge development;
- How the theory stands up to testing.

Within each of these, criteria have been highlighted which will act as a guide through the analysis process.

I would caution that there are no correct answers to many of the questions which analysis will uncover. You could prefix each of the above criteria with the words 'should a theory be . . .'. Such an analysis will undoubtedly create a great deal of information about the theorist, the theory and its usefulness. However, keep in mind the possibility that perhaps all theories should not adhere to all of the criteria for analysis and evaluation.

Apart from the reference list and an appendix you have now reached the end of the book. I hope you have enjoyed reading it. It should provide you with up-to-date knowledge on theoretical terminology, on the philosophical basis for knowing in nursing, on how concepts can be analysed, on what nursing theory is and on how to select, apply and test theory.

Compared to established professions such as medicine, architecture and the law, nursing has come a long way in a very short space of time. In the 1960s in the US, Henderson collected all the published nursing research available and it filled two slim volumes. Nursing research in the UK took a little longer to build a body of literature. From Chapter 4 you will recall that contemporary theorising has a similar vintage. We have come from being in a pre-paradigmatic phase of development to having several competing paradigms.

All nurses have a role to play in the future of the discipline: this role should involve strengthening the relationship between practice, theory and research. Part of this will involve contributing to general health care theories by working in equal partnership with patients and other professionals. If nurses fail to play their part we will be stumbling backwards into the twenty-first century.

Appendix
Summary of the main nursing theories and their metaparadigm components

Theorist	'Person'	'Nursing'	'Health'	'Environment'
Roper, Logan and Tierney (1980)	Unfragmented whole who carries out, or is assisted in carrying out, activities which contribute to the process of living.	A profession whose focus is to help the patient prevent, solve, alleviate, or cope with problems associated with the activities of living.	The optimum level of independence in each activity of living which enables the individual to function at his or her maximum capacity.	Circumstances which may impinge upon people as they travel along the life-span and cause movement to dependence or independence.
Wiedenbach (1964)	A functionally competent being, able to determine if a need for help is being experienced.	A helping art which uses a unique blend of thoughts and feelings and overt actions in relation to an individual who is in need of help.	A nurse's concern for the patient is related to his or her health.	That which may produce an obstacle which may result in a need for help.
Orem (1995)	Functional integrated whole with a motivation to achieve self-care.	A human service related to the patient's need and ability to undertake self-care and to help him or her sustain health, recover from disease and injury or cope with their effects.	A state of wholeness or integrity of the individual, his or her parts and modes of functioning.	A subcomponent of the person, and with the person forms an integrated system related to self-care.
Minshull, Ross and Turner (1986)	A holistic individual having interdependent physical, psycho-social, spiritual and social needs.	Supports, enables or helps the individual, either directly or indirectly, to meet their need to achieve maximum wellness and independence.	A relatively stable state of maximum wellness which equates with independence.	That area in which the individual functions.

Rogers (1980)	A unified whole; a unique unitary field of energy that manifests characteristics that are more than and different from the sum of their parts.	A learned profession with compassionate concern for maintaining and promoting health, preventing illness, caring for and rehabilitating the sick and disabled.	Defined by cultures and individuals to denote behaviours that are of high value and low value.	A four-dimensional negatrophic energy field identified by pattern and organisation, and encompassing all that is outside any given field.
Henderson (1966)	Biological human beings with inseparable mind and body who share certain fundamental human needs.	A profession which assists the person, sick or well, in the performance of those activities contributing to health or its reccovery (or to a peaceful death); that the person would perform if he or she had the strength, will or knowledge.	The ability to function independently regarding fourteen fundamental activities of daily living.	That which may act in a positive or negative way upon the patient.
Johnson (1959)	A behavioural system having eight sub-systems which are interrelated and interdependent.	A professional discipline giving a socially valued service which focuses on the individual who is attempting to maintain or re-establish equilibrium.	An elusive state determined by psychological, social and physiological factors which is held as a desired value by all the health professions.	That which is external to the person but from which he or she receives sustenal needs.
Roy (1970)	A bio-psycho-social being who presents as an integrated whole.	A socially valued service whose goal is to promote a positive adaptation to the stimuli and stresses encountered by the patient.	The adaptation of the person to stimuli on a continuous line between wellness and illness.	Both internal and external; from the environment, the person is subject to stresses.

Theorist	'Person'	'Nursing'	'Health'	'Environment'
Neuman (1982)	A total person having physiological, psychological, socio-cultural and developmental influences.	A unique profession which can purposefully intervene at primary, secondary or tertiary prevention levels.	A varying state of wellness and illness which is influenced by physiological, psychological, socio-cultural and developmental factors.	Both internal and external with the person maintaining varying degrees of harmony between both.
Fitzpatrick (1982)	An open system, a unified whole, characterised by basic human rhythms.	A science and a profession which has as its central concern the meaning attached to life and health.	A continuously developing characteristic of humans: awareness and meaningfulness of life and full life potential.	An open system in continuous interaction with the person.
Parse (1981)	A synergistic open being co-extensive with the universe and free to choose in situations.	Science and an art focusing on man as a living unit.	A process of becoming, as experienced by the person.	Co-constituted becoming in mutual simultaneous energy exchange with the person.
Newman (1979)	An energy field that is part of the life process.	Nursing assists individuals to utilise their own resources to attain higher levels of consciousness.	A fusion of disease and non-disease that is a basic pattern unique to the person as he or she evolves towards expanded consciousness.	An energy field that is part of the life process, that which is outside any given human field.
Travelbee (1966)	Unique irreplaceable individuals who are always in the process of learning, evolving or changing.	An interpersonal process which assists the individual, family or community to prevent or cope with illness/suffering and find meaning and hope in these experiences.	A subjective state that is determined in accord with each person's appraisal of his or her physical, emotional or spiritual status.	The arena where man experiences the full range of the human condition.

Peplau (1952)	A unique self-system composed of biochemical, physiological and interpersonal characteristics.	A significant therapeutic interpersonal process which acts as a maturing force and an educative instrument.	Forward movements of personality and other ongoing human processes in the direction of creative, constructive, productive personal and community living.	Microcosms of significant others and interpersonal situations with whom the person interacts.
Levine (1966)	A living being who interacts with his or her environment and responds by means of change by means of adapting.	A process of human interaction which incorporates scientific principles in the use of the nursing process.	A pattern of adaptive change.	Both internal (physiological) and external (perceptual, operational, conceptual) components.
Patterson and Zderad (1976)	An incarnate being always becoming in relation to persons and things in a world of time and space.	An intersubjective transaction between patient and nurse related to the health–illness quality of living.	More than just freedom from disease.	The person's inner world (a biased and shaded reality), and the real world (persons and things in time and space).
King (1971)	An open system interacting with the environment, each permitting an exchange of matter, energy and information through permeable boundaries.	A process of interaction between nurse and client whereby each perceives the other and the situation: and through communication they set goals, explore means, and agree on means to achieve goals.	A dynamic state in the life cycle, which implies continuous adaptation to stresses through optimal use of one's resources to achieve maximum potential for daily living.	An open system permitting an exchange of matter, energy and information with human beings through permeable boundaries.

Theorist	'Person'	'Nursing'	'Health'	'Environment'
Orlando (1961)	A behaving human organism.	Interaction with a patient with a need which involves patient validation with the needed and the help provided in order to improve the patient's health.	Mental and physical comfort, a sense of adequacy and well-being.	Time and place – the context of the nursing situation.
Riehl (1974)	One who has intrinsic value and who is constantly striving to make sense of the situation in which he finds himself.	A professional service involving direct and personal ministrations to individuals, families and groups wherever they are when health needs arise.	An optimum state of health is considered as a state of wholeness.	Environment is dynamic with many interesting forces serving as a constraint impinging on and influencing the person's state of health.

References

Note: In general the most recent edition of a work has been cited, but details and, where appropriate, an entry for previous editions are given where the work has been updated.

Abdellah, F.G., Beland, I.L., Martin, A. and Matheney, R.V. (1960), *Patient Centred Approaches to Nursing*, New York: Macmillan.

Adam, E. (1992), 'Contemporary conceptualisations of nursing: philosophies or science?', in Kikuchi, J.F. and Simmons, H. (eds), *Philosophic Inquiry in Nursing*, Newbury Park: Sage.

Adam, E.T. (1975), 'A conceptual model for nursing', *The Canadian Nurse*, 71: 40–3.

—— (1980), *To Be a Nurse*, New York: W.B. Saunders.

—— (1983), 'Frontiers of nursing in the 21st century: development of models and theories on the concept of nursing', *Journal of Advanced Nursing*, 8(1): 41 5.

Aggleton, P. and Chalmers, H. (1986), *Nursing Models and the Nursing Process*, Basingstoke: Macmillan.

Aggleton, P.J. and Chalmers, H.A. (1987), 'Nursing research, nursing theory and the nursing process', *Journal of Advanced Nursing*, 12(5): 573–81.

Aggleton, P. and Chalmers, C. (1990), 'Nursing models: model future', *Nursing Times*, 86(3): 41–3.

Allen. M.N. and Hayes, P. (1989), 'Models of nursing: implications for research in nursing', in Akinsanya, J. (ed.), *Recent Advances in Nursing*, 24, Edinburgh: Churchill Livingstone.

Altschul, A.T. (1980), 'The care of the mentally disordered: three approaches', *Nursing Times*, 76(11): 452–4.

Arets, J. and Slevin, O. (1995), 'European nursing models', in Slevin, O. (ed.), *The Theoretical Basis of Nursing*, Edinburgh: Campion Press.

Argyris, C. and Schon, D. (1974), *Theory in Practice: Increasing Professional Effectiveness*, London: Jossey-Bass.

Armitage, P. (1990), 'An evaluation of primary nursing and the role of the nurse preceptor in changing long-term mental health care', unpublished Ph.D. thesis, University of Wales.

Baldwin, S. (1983), 'Nursing models in special hospital settings', *Journal of Advanced Nursing*, 8: 473–6.

Barber, P. (1986), 'The psychiatric nurse's failure therapeutically to nurture', *Nursing Practice*, 1(3): 138–41.

Barker, P.J. (1991), 'Finding common ground', *Nursing Times*, 87(2): 37–8.

Barnum, B.J.S. (1990), *Nursing Theory: Analysis, Application, Evaluation* (3rd edn), Philadelphia: Little Brown.

Batey, M.V. (1971), 'Conceptualizing the research process', *Nursing Research*, 20(4): 296–301.

Beck, C.T. (1985), 'Theoretical frameworks', cited in *Nursing Research* from January 1974–June 1985, *Nurse Educator*, 10(6): 36–8.

Beckstrand, J. (1980), 'A critique of several conceptions of practice theory in nursing', *Research in Nursing and Health*, 3(2): 69–80.

Benner, P. (1984), 'Uncovering the knowledge embedded in clinical practice', in Benner, P. (ed.), *From Novice to Expert*, New York: Addison Wesley.

Biley, F. (1991), 'The divide between theory and practice', *Nursing*, 4(29): 30–3.

Bishop, S.M. (1986), 'History and philosophy of science', in Marriner, A. (ed.), *Nursing Theorists and their Work*, St Louis: C.V. Mosby.

Blumer, H. (1969), *Symbolic Interactionism: Perspective and Method*, Englewood Cliffs: Prentice Hall.

Bogdanovic, A. (1989), 'Non-verbal communication', *Nursing Times*, 85(1): 27–8.

Bohny, B. (1980), 'Theory development for a nursing science', *Nursing Forum*, 19(1): 50–67.

Boore, J.R.P. (1978), *A Prescription for Recovery*, London: Royal College of Nursing.

Botha, M.E. (1989), 'Theory development in perspective: the role of conceptual frameworks and models in theory development', *Journal of Advanced Nursing*, 14: 49–55.

Boud, D., Keogh, R. and Walker, D. (1985), *Reflection: Turning Experience into Learning*, London: Kogan Page.

Boykin, A. and Schoenhofer, S. (1993), *Nursing as Caring: A Model for Transforming Practice*, New York: National League of Nursing.

Brent, K. (1993), 'Perspective on critical and feminist theory in development nursing praxis', *Journal of Professional Nursing*, 9(5): 296–303.

Brett, J.L.L. (1987), 'Use of nursing practice research findings', *Nursing Research*, 36(6): 344–9.

Brewster, M., Cook, M. and Woodward, S. (1991), 'Standard care plan system: critical but stable', paper presented at the Quality Assurance Network Conference, Oxford.

Bronowski, J. (1965), *Science and Human Values*, New York: Julian Messner.

Brown, M.I. (1964), 'Research in the development of nursing theory: the importance of a theoretical framework in nursing research', *Nursing Research*, 13(2): 109–12.

Bryar, R.M. (1995), *Theory for Midwifery Practice*, London: Macmillan.

Buber, M. (1962), *Ten Rungs: Hasidic Sayings*, New York: Schocken.

Burnard, P. (1990), 'Thoughts about theories', *Nursing Standard*, 4(21): 47.

Capers, C.F. (1986), 'Using nursing models to guide nursing practice: key questions', *Journal of Nursing Administration*, 16(11): 40–3.

Carper, B.A. (1978), 'Fundamental patterns of knowing in nursing', *Advances in Nursing Science*, 1(1): 13–23.

—— (1992), 'Philosophical inquiry in nursing: an application', in Kikuchi, J.F. and Simmons, H. (eds), *Philosophic Inquiry in Nursing*, Newbury Park: Sage.

Cash, K. (1990), 'Nursing models and the idea of nursing', *International Journal of Nursing Studies*, 27(3): 249–56.

Castledine, G. (1986), 'A stress adaptation model', in Kershaw, B. and Salvage, J. (eds), *Models for Nursing*, Chichester: John Wiley & Sons.

Chalmers, H. (ed.) (1988), *Cardiovascular and Respiratory Care: Choosing a Model Series*, London: Edward Arnold.

Chalmers, H. (ed.) (1989), 'Theories and models of nursing and the nursing process', in Akinsanya, J.A. (ed.), *Theories and Models of Nursing*, Edinburgh: Churchill Livingstone.

Chambers, M. (1995), 'Learning psychiatric nursing skills: the contribution of the ward environment', unpublished D.Phil. thesis, University of Ulster.

Chapman, C.M. (1985), *Theory of Nursing: Practical Application*, London: Harper & Row.

Chapman, P. (1990), 'A critical perspective', in Salvage, J. and Kershaw, B. (eds), *Models for Nursing 2*, London: Scutari Press.

Chavasse, J. (1987), 'A comparison of three models of nursing', *Nurse Education Today*, 7(4): 177–86.

Chin, R. and Benne, K.D. (1976), 'General strategies for effecting changes', in Bennis, W.G., Benne, K.D., Chin, R. and Corey, K.E. (eds), *The Planning of Change* (3rd edn), New York: Holt, Rinehart & Winston.

Chinn, P. and Jacobs, M.K. (1987), *Theory and Nursing: A Systematic Approach* (2nd edn; 1st edn 1983), St Louis: C.V. Mosby.

Chinn, P. and Kramer, M.K. (1991), *Theory and Nursing: A Systematic Approach* (3rd edn), St Louis: C.V. Mosby.

Chinn, P. and Kramer, M.K. (1995), *Theory and Nursing: A Systematic Approach* (4th edn), St Louis: C.V. Mosby.

Clare, A. (1976), *Psychiatry in Dissent*, London: Tavistock.

Clark, J. (1986), 'A model for health visiting', in Kershaw, B. and Salvage, J. (eds), *Models for Nursing*. Chichester: John Wiley & Sons.

Clarke, M. (1986), 'Action and reflection: practice and theory in nursing', *Journal of Advanced Nursing*, 11: 3–11.

Clinton, M. (1981), 'Training psychiatric nurses: a sociological study of the problems of integrating theory and practice', unpublished Ph.D. thesis, University of East Anglia.

Cody, W. K. (1994), 'Nursing theory-guided practice: what it is and what it is not', *Nursing Science Quarterly*, 7(4): 144–5.

—— (1995), 'All about those paradigms: many in the universe, two in nursing', *Nursing Science Quarterly*, 8(4): 144–7.

Collister, B. (1988), *Psychiatric Nursing: Person to Person*, London: Edward Arnold.

Craig, S.L. (1980), 'Theory development and its relevance for nursing', *Journal of Advanced Nursing*, 5: 349–55.

Denyes, M.J., O'Connor, N.A., Oakley, D. and Ferguson, S. (1989), 'Integrating nursing theory, practice and research through collaborative research', *Journal of Advanced Nursing*, 14: 141–5.

Department of Health (1994), *Working in Partnership. The Report from the Mental Health Review Team*, London: HMSO.

Dewey, J. (1933), *How We Think*, Boston: D.C. Heath.

Dickoff, J. and James, P. (1968), 'A theory of theories: a position paper', *Nursing Research*, 17(3): 197–203.

Dickoff, J. and James, P. (1971), 'Clarity to what end?' *Nursing Research*, 20(6): 499–502.

Dickoff, J. and James, P. (1982), 'Towards a cultivated but decisive pluralism in nursing', in McGee, M. (ed.), *Theoretical Pluralism in Nursing Science*, Ottawa: University of Ottawa Press (pp. 9–83).

Dickoff, J. and James, P. (1992), 'Correspondence', in Nicholl, L. (ed.), *Perspectives on Nursing Theory* (2nd edn), New York: Lippincott.

Diers, D. (1979), *Research in Nursing Practice*, Philadelphia: J.B. Lippincott Co.

Donaldson, S.K. and Crowley, D. (1978), 'The discipline of nursing', *Nursing Outlook*, 26(2): 113–20.

Draper, P. (1991), 'The ideal and the real: some thoughts on the theoretical developments in British nursing', *Nurse Education Today*, 11: 292–4.

Duldt, B. and Griffin, K. (1985), *Theoretical Perspectives for Nursing*, Boston: Little Brown & Co.

Dyer, S. (1990), 'Nursing models: teamwork for personal patient care', *Nursing the Elderly*, 1(5): 28–30.

Ellis, R. (1968), 'Characteristics of significant theories', *Nursing Research*, 17(3): 217–22.

—— (1969), 'The practitioner as theorist', *American Journal of Nursing*, 69: 1434–8.

—— (1970), 'Values and vicissitudes of the scientist nurse', *Nursing Research*, 19(5): 440–5.

Emden, C. (1991), 'Ways of knowing in nursing', in Gray, G. and Pratt, R. (eds), *Towards a Discipline of Nursing*, Edinburgh: Churchill Livingstone.

Engel, G.L. (1977), 'The need for a new medical model: a challenge for biomedicine', *Science*, 196 (4286): 129–36.

Engstrom, J.L. (1984), 'Problems in the development, use and testing of nursing theory', *Journal of Nurse Education*, 23(6): 245–51.

Erickson, H., Tomlin, E, and Swain, M. (1983), *Modelling and Role Modelling*, Lexington: Pine Press.

Eysenck, H.J. (1971), 'A mish-mash of theories', *International Journal of Psychiatry*, 109: 12–18.

Farmer, E. (1986), 'Exploring the issues', in Kershaw, B. and Salvage, J. (eds), *Models for Nursing*, Chichester: John Wiley & Sons.

Fawcett, J. (1980), 'A framework for analysis and evaluation of conceptual models of nursing', *Nurse Educator*, 5(12): 12–14.

—— (1989), *Analysis and Evaluation of Conceptual Models of Nursing* (2nd edn; 1st edn 1984), Philadelphia: F.A. Davis.

—— (1990), 'Preparation for Caesarean childbirth: derivation of a nursing intervention from the Roy adaptation model', *Journal of Advanced Nursing*, 15: 1418–25.

—— (1992), 'Contemporary conceptualisations of nursing: philosophy or science?', in Kikuchi, J.F. and Simmons, H. (eds), *Philosophic Inquiry in Nursing*, Newbury Park: Sage.

—— (1995), *Analysis and Evaluation of Theories of Nursing*, Philadelphia: F.A. Davis.

Fawcett, J. and Carino, C. (1989), 'Hallmarks of success in nursing practice', *Advances in Nursing Science*, 11(4): 1–8.

Fawcett, J. and Downs, F.S. (1992), *The Relationship of Theory and Research* (2nd edn), Philadelphia: F.A. Davis.

Feyerabend, P. (1975), *Against Method: Outline of an Anarchistic Theory of Knowledge*, London: New Left.

—— (1977), 'Consolidation for the specialist', in Lakatos, I. and Musgrave, A. (eds), *Criticism and the Growth of Knowledge*, Cambridge: Cambridge University Press.

Field, P.A. and Morse, J.M. (1985), *Nursing Research: The Application of Qualitative Approaches*, London: Croom Helm.

Firlit, S.L. (1990), 'Nursing theory and nursing practice: do they connect?, in McCloskey, G. and Grace, H. (eds), *Current Issues in Nursing*, St Louis: C.V. Mosby.

Fitzpatrick, J.J. (1982) 'Fitzpatrick's model', in Fitzpatrick, J.J. *et al.*, *Nursing Models: Application to Psychiatric Mental Health Nursing*, Maryland: Brady Co.

Fitzpatrick, J.J. and Whall, A.L. (1996), *Conceptual Models of Nursing: Analysis and Application* (3rd edn; 1st edn 1983; 2nd edn 1989), Connecticut: Appleton & Lange.

Fogel-Keck, J (1994), 'Terminology of theory development', in Marriner-Tomey, A. (ed.), *Nursing Theorists and their Work* (3rd edn), St Louis: C.V. Mosby.

Folta, J.R. (1971), 'Obfuscation or clarification: a reaction to Walker's concept of nursing theory', *Nursing Research*, 20(6): 496–9.

Forchuk, C. (1991), 'Peplau's theory: concepts and their relations', *Nursing Science Quarterly*, 4: 54–60.

Fraser, M. (1996), *Using Conceptual Nursing in Practice: A Research-based Approach* (2nd edn; 1st edn 1990), London: Harper & Row.

Fretwell, S.E. (1985), *Freedom to Change*, London: RCN.

Freud, S. (1949), *An Outline of Psychoanalysis*, New York: W.W. Norton.

Friend, B. (1990), 'Working at health', *Nursing Times*, 86(16): 21.

Fry, S.T. (1992), 'Neglect of philosophical enquiry in nursing: cause and effect', in Kikuchi, J.F. and Simmons, H. (eds), *Philosophic Inquiry in Nursing*, Newbury Park: Sage.

Gadow, S. (1990), 'Response to "personal knowing: evolving research and practice"', *Scholarly Inquiry in Nursing Practice*, 4(2): 167–70.

George, J. (ed.) (1975), *Nursing Theories: The Base for Professional Practice* (1st edn), Englewood Cliffs: Prentice Hall.

—— (1985), *Nursing Theories: The Base for Professional Practice* (2nd edn), Englewood Cliffs: Prentice Hall.

—— (1995), *Nursing Theories: The Base for Professional Practice* (4th edn), Englewood Cliffs: Prentice Hall.

Girot, E. (1990), 'Discussing nursing theory', *Senior Nurse*, 10(6): 16–19.

Glaser, B. and Strauss, A. (1967), *The Discovery of Grounded Theory*, Chicago: Aldine.

Goffman, E. (1961), *Asylums: Essays on the Social Situations of Mental Patients and Other Inmates*, Harmondsworth: Pelican.

Goodridge, D. and Hack, B. (1996), 'Assessing the congruence of nursing models with organisational culture: a quality improvement perspective', *Journal of Nursing Care Quality*, 10(2): 41–8.

Gordon, D.R. (1984), 'Research application: identifying the use and misuse of formal models in nursing practice', in Benner, P. (ed.), *From Novice to Expert*, New York: Addison Wesley.

Gortner, S.R. (1993), 'Nursing's syntax revisited: a critique of philosophies said to influence nursing theories', *International Journal of Nursing Studies*, 30(6): 477–88.

Gottlieb, L. and Rowat, K. (1987), 'The McGill model of nursing: a practice-derived model', *Advances in Nursing Science*, 9(4): 51–61.

Gould, D. (1989), 'Teaching theories and models of nursing: implications for a common foundation programme for nurses', in Akinsanya, J.A. (ed.), *Theories and Models of Nursing*, Edinburgh: Churchill Livingstone.

Grahame (1987), 'Backchat', *Nursing Times*, 83(16): 22.

Gray, J. and Forsstrom, S. (1992), 'Generating theory from practice: the reflective technique', in Gray, G. and Pratt, R. (eds), *Towards a Discipline of Nursing*, Edinburgh: Churchill Livingstone.

Greaves, F. (1984), *Nurse Education and the Curriculum: A Curricular Model*, London: Croom Helm.

Green, C. (1985), 'An overview of the value of nursing models in relation to education', *Nurse Education Today*, 5: 267–71.

—— (1988), 'The development of a conceptual model for mental handicap nursing practice in the UK', *Nurse Education Today*, 8: 9–17.

Greenhalgh, C. & Co. (1994), *The Interface between Junior Doctors and Nurses*, London: Greenhalgh Consultants & Co.

Habermas, J. (1971), *Knowledge and Human Interests*, Boston: Beacon Press.

Hagemeier, D. and Hunt, C. (1979), 'Do new graduates use conceptual frameworks?', *Nursing Outlook*, Aug.: 545–8.

Hall, B.A. (1993), 'The theory–research–practice triad', *Nursing Science Quarterly*, 6(1): 10–11.

Hall, L. (1959), *Nursing – What Is It?*, Virginia: Virginia State Nurses Association.

—— (1966), 'Another view of nursing care and quality', in Straub,

K.M. and Parker, K.S. (eds), *Continuity in Client Care: The Role of Nursing*, Washington: Catholic University Press.

Haller, K.B., Reynolds, M.A. and Horsley, J.A. (1979), 'Developing research-based innovation protocols: process criteria, and issues', *Research in Nursing and Health*, 2: 45–51.

Hardy, L.K. (1982), 'Nursing models and research – a restricting view?', *Journal of Advanced Nursing*, 7: 447–51.

—— (1986), 'Janforum: identifying the place of theoretical frameworks in an evolving discipline', *Journal of Advanced Nursing* 11: 103–7.

Hardy, M.E. (1978), 'Perspectives on nursing theory', *Advances in Nursing Science*, 1(1): 27–48.

—— (1991), 'Theories: components, development, evaluation', in Nichol, L.H. (ed.), *Perspectives on Nursing Theory*, New York: J.B. Lippincott.

Hawkett, S. (1989), 'A model marriage', *Nursing Times*, 85(1): 61–2.

Henderson, V. (1966), *The Nature of Nursing: A Definition and its Implications for Practice, Education and Research*, London: Collier Macmillan.

Henderson, V. and Harmer, B. (1955), *Textbook of the Principles and Practices of Nursing* (5th edn), New York: Macmillan.

Hersey, P. and Blanchard, K.H. (1977), *Management of Organizational Behaviour: Utilizing Human Resources* (3rd edn), Englewood Cliffs: Prentice Hall.

Hinshaw, A.S. (1989), 'Nursing science: the challenge to develop knowledge', *Nursing Science Quarterly*, 2(4): 162–71.

Hoch, C.C. (1987), 'Assessing delivery of nursing care', *Journal of Gerontological Nursing*, 13(1): 10–17.

Holden, R.J. (1990), 'Models, muddles and medicine', *International Journal of Nursing Studies*, 27(3): 223–34.

Houlihan, P.J. (1986), 'The marketing of nursing jargon', *The Canadian Nurse*, Feb.: 21–2.

Huch, M.H. (1995), 'Nursing and the next millennium', *Nursing Science Quarterly*, 8(1): 38–44.

Hunink, G. (1995), *A Study Guide to Nursing Theories*, Edinburgh: Campion Press.

Hunt, J. (1981), 'Indicators for nursing practice', *Journal of Advanced Nursing*, 16: 89–114.

Husserl, E. (1962), *Ideas: General Introduction to Pure Phenomenology* (trans. R.B. Goodman), New York: Collier.

Jackson, M. (1986), 'On maps and models', *Senior Nurse*, 5(4): 24–6.

Jacobson, S. (1987), 'Studying and using conceptual models of nursing', *Image: The Journal of Nurse Scholarship*, 19(2): 78–83.

Jacox, A.K. (1974), 'Theory construction in nursing: an overview', *Nursing Research*, 23(1): 4–13.

Jacox, A.K. and Webster, G. (1992), 'Competing theories of science', in Nicoll, L. (ed.), *Perspectives on Nursing Theory* (2nd edn), New York: J.B. Lippincott.

Jennings, B.M. and Meleis, A.I. (1988), 'Nursing theory and administrative practice', *Advances in Nursing Science*, 10(3): 56–69.

Jensen, A.R. (1973), 'Race, intelligence and genetics: the differences are real', *Psychology Today*, 12: 80–6.

Johnson, D.E. (1959), 'The nature of a science of nursing', *Nursing Outlook*, 7: 291–4.

—— (1968), 'Theory in nursing: borrowed and unique', *Nursing Research*, 17(3): 206–9.

Johnson, M. (1983), 'Some aspects of the relation between theory and research in nursing', *Journal of Advanced Nursing*, 8: 21–8.

Johnson, N. and Baumann, A. (1992), 'Selecting a nursing model for psychiatric nursing: a process-oriented approach', *Journal of Psychosocial Nursing*, 30(4): 7–12.

Jones, A. (1990), 'The value of models in district nursing', in Salvage, J. and Kershaw, B. (eds), *Models for Nursing 2*, London: Scutari Press.

Jukes, M. (1988), 'Nursing model or psychological assessment?', *Senior Nurse*, 8(11): 8–10.

Kant, I. (1953), *Prolegomena to any Future Metaphysics* (trans. P.G. Lucas), Manchester: University of Manchester Press.

Kaplan, A. (1964), *The Conduct of Inquiry: Methodology for Behavioural Sciences*, Scranton: P.A. Chandler.

Kemmis, S. (1985), 'Action research and the politics of reflection', in Boud, D., Keogh, R. and Walker, D. (eds), (1985), *Reflection: Turning Experience into Learning*, London: Kogan Page.

Kemp, V.A. (1990), 'Themes in theory development', in Chaska, N.L. (ed.), *The Nursing Profession: Turning Points*, St Louis: C.V. Mosby.

Kerlinger, F.N.B. (1986), *Foundations of Behavioural Research* (3rd edn), New York: Holt, Rinehart & Winston.

Kershaw, B. (1986), 'Introduction', in Kershaw, B. and Salvage, J. (eds), *Models for Nursing*, Chichester: John Wiley & Sons.

—— (1990), 'Towards 2000', in Salvage, J. and Kershaw, B. (eds), *Models for Nursing 2*, London: Scutari Press.

Kershaw, B. and Salvage, J. (eds) (1986), *Models for Nursing*, Chichester: John Wiley & Sons.

Kesey K. (1962), *One Flew Over the Cuckoo's Nest*, London: Pan Books.

Keyzer, D.M. (1985), 'Learning contracts: the trained nurse and the implementation of the nursing process: comparative case studies in the management of knowledge and change in nursing practice', unpublished Ph.D. thesis, Institute of Education, University of London.

Kikuchi, J.F. (1992), 'Nursing questions that science cannot answer', in Kikuchi, J.F. and Simmons, H. (eds), *Philosophic Inquiry in Nursing*, Newbury Park: Sage.

Kikuchi, J.F. and Simmons, H. (eds) (1992), *Philosophic Inquiry in Nursing*, Newbury Park: Sage.

Kikuchi, J.F. and Simmons, H. (eds) (1994), *Developing a Philosophy of Nursing*, Newbury Park: Sage.

Kim, H.S. (1983), *The Nature of Theoretical Thinking in Nursing*, Norwalk, Conn.: Appleton–Century–Crofts.

—— (1989), 'Theoretical thinking in nursing', in Akinsanya, J. (ed.), *Recent Advances in Nursing*, 24, Edinburgh: Churchill Livingstone.

—— (1994), 'Practice theories in nursing and a science of nursing practice', *Scholarly Inquiry for Nursing Practice*, 8(2): 145–58.

King, I. (1968), 'A conceptual frame of reference for nursing', *Nursing Research*, 17(1): 27–31.

—— (1971), *Towards a Theory of Nursing*, New York: John Wiley & Sons.

King, I. (1981), *A Theory of Nursing: Systems, Concepts, Process*, New York: John Wiley.

Kirby, C. and Slevin, O. (1995), cited in Arets, J. and Slevin, O., 'European nursing models', in Slevin, O, *The Theoretical Basis of Nursing*, Edinburgh: Campion Press.

Kitson, A.L. (1984), 'A study of geriatric wards, their patients and nursing staff in Northern Ireland', unpublished paper, University of Ulster.

Koziel-McCain, J. and Meave, M.K. (1993), 'Nursing theory in perspective', *Nursing Outlook*, 41(2): 79–81.

Kristjanson, L.J., Tamblyn, R. and Kuypers, J.A. (1987), 'A model to guide development and application of multiple nursing theories', *Journal of Advanced Nursing*, 12: 523–9.

Kuhn, T.S. (1962), *The Structure of Scientific Revolutions* (1st edn), Chicago: University of Chicago Press.

—— (1970), *The Structure of Scientific Revolutions* (2nd edn), Chicago: University of Chicago Press.

—— (1977), *The Structure of Scientific Revolutions* (3rd edn), Chicago: University of Chicago Press.

Lancaster, J. and Lancaster, W. (1982), *The Nurse as a Change Agent*, St Louis: C.V. Mosby.

Laudan, L. (1977), *Progress and its Problems: Towards a Theory of Scientific Growth*, Berkeley: University of California Press.

Leddy, S. and Pepper, J.M. (1989), *Conceptual Bases of Professional Nursing*, Philadelphia: J.B. Lippincott.

Leininger, M.M. (1978), *Transcultural Nursing: Concepts, Theories, and Practices*, New York: John Wiley & Sons.

—— (1981), *Caring: An Essential Human Need*, Thorofare: Stack.

Lerheim, K. (1991), 'Nursing science – does it make a difference?', *International Nursing Review*, 38(3): 73–8.

Levine, M.E. (1966), 'Adaptation and assessment: a rationale for nursing intervention', *American Journal of Nursing*, 66(11): 2450–3.

—— (1994), 'Some further thoughts on the ethics of nursing rhetoric', in Kikuchi, J.F. and Simmons, H. (eds), *Developing a Philosophy of Nursing*, Thousand Oaks: Sage.

—— (1995), 'The rhetoric of nursing theory', *Image: The Journal of Nurse Scholarship*, 27(1): 11–14.

Lewin, K. (1951), *Field Theory in Social Science*, Connecticut: Greenwood Press.

Lindsay, B. (1990), 'The gap between theory and practice', *Nursing Standard*, 5(4): 34–5.

Lippitt, G. (1973), *Visualising Change: Model Building and the Change Process*, La Jolla: University Associates Inc.

Lister, P. (1987), 'The misunderstood model', *Nursing Times*, 83(41): 40–2.

Loughlin, M. (1988), 'Modelled, muddled and befuddled', *Nursing Times*, 84(5): 30–1.

Luker, K. (1987), 'Applying models of nursing in the community', paper read at Second International Primary Health Care Conference, London.

—— (1988), 'Debate 1: this house believes that nursing models provide a useful tool in the management of patient care', in Pritchard, A.P. (ed.), *Proceedings of the Fifth International Conference on Cancer Nursing*, London: Macmillan Press.

Lynn, G. (1996), 'Intelligence and gender', unpublished paper, University of Ulster.

McCance, T. (1996), 'Concept analysis of caring', unpublished D.Phil. thesis, University of Ulster.

McFarlane, J.K. (1982), 'Nursing: a paradigm of caring', unpublished conference paper, Ethical Issues in Caring, University of Manchester.

—— (1986a), 'Looking to the future', in Kershaw, B. and Salvage, J. (eds), *Models for Nursing*, Chichester: John Wiley & Sons.

—— (1986b), 'The value of models of care', in Kershaw, B. and Salvage, J. (eds), *Models for Nursing*, Chichester: John Wiley & Sons.

McGee, M. (1994), 'Eclecticism in nursing philosophy: problem or solution?', in Kikuchi, J.F. and Simmons, H. (eds), *Developing a Philosophy of Nursing*, Thousand Oaks: Sage.

McKenna, G. (1993), 'Unique theory: is it essential in the development of a science of nursing?', *Nurse Education Today*, 13: 121–7.

McKenna, H.P. (1989), 'The selection by ward managers of an appropriate nursing model for long-stay psychiatric patient care', *Journal of Advanced Nursing*, 14: 762–75.

—— (1990), 'A pill for every ill', *Nursing Times*, 86(10): 28–31.

—— (1992), 'The selection and evaluation of a nursing model in long-stay psychiatric wards', unpublished D.Phil. thesis, University of Ulster.

—— (1993), 'Research and destroy', *Nursing Standard*, 8(12): 50–1.

—— (1994a), *Nursing Theories and Quality of Care*, Aldershot: Avebury.

—— (1994b), 'The attitudes of traditional and undergraduate nursing students towards nursing models: a comparative survey', *Journal of Advanced Nursing*, 19(3): 527–37.

—— (with Parahoo, K.A. and Boore, J.R.P.) (1995), 'The evaluation of a nursing model for long-stay psychiatric patient care: Part 1, literature review and methodology', and 'Part 2, presentation and discussion of findings', *International Journal of Nursing Studies*, 31(1): 79–94 and 95–113.

McQuiston C.M. and Webb, A.A. (1995), *Foundations of Nursing Theory: Contributions of Twelve Key Theorists*, Thousand Oaks: Sage.

Maloney, E. (1984), 'Theoretical approaches', in Beck, C.A., Rawlings, R.P. and Williams, S.R. (eds), *Mental Health Psychiatric Nursing: A Holistic Life Cycle Approach*, St Louis: C.V. Mosby.

Mansfield, E. (1980), 'A conceptual framework for psychiatric mental health care nursing', *Journal of Psychiatric Nursing and Mental Health Services*, 18(4): 34–41.

Marriner-Tomey, A. (1994), *Nursing Theorists and Their Work* (3rd edn), St Louis: C.V. Mosby.

Maslow, A.H. (1954), *Motivation and Personality*, New York: Harper & Row.

Mason, T. and Chanley, M. (1990), 'Nursing models in a special hospital: a critical analysis of efficacy', *Journal of Advanced Nursing*, 15: 667–73.

Masterman, M. (1970), 'The nature of a paradigm', in Lakatos, I. and Musgrave, A. (eds), *Criticism and the Growth of Knowledge*, Cambridge: Cambridge University Press.

Meave, M.K. (1994), 'The carrier bag theory of nursing practice', *Advances in Nursing Science*, 16(4): 9–22.

Meleis, A.I. (1985), *Theoretical Nursing: Development and Progress*, Philadelphia: Lippincott.

Meleis, A.I. (1991), *Theoretical Nursing: Development and Progress* (2nd edn), Philadelphia: Lippincott.

—— (1995), 'Development of theory from practice', workshop presentation in Kristianstad, Sweden, March.

Melia, K. (1990), 'Nursing models: enhancing or inhibiting practice?' *Nursing Standard*, 5(11): 34–5.

Menzies, I.E.P. (1960), 'A case study in the functioning of social systems as a defence against anxiety: a report of a study of the nursing service of a general hospital', *Human Relations*, 13(2): 95–121.

Merchant, J. (1991), 'Task allocation: a case of resistance to change', *Nursing Practice*, 4(2): 16–18.

Merton, R.K. (1968), *Social Theory and Social Structure*, New York: Free Press.

Metcalf, C. (1982), 'A study of a change in the method of organising the delivery of nursing care in a ward of a maternity hospital', unpublished D.Phil. thesis, University of Manchester.

Midgley, C. (1988), 'The use of models for nursing within midwifery training hospitals in England', unpublished paper, Huddersfield Polytechnic.

Miller, A.E. (1985), 'The relationship between nursing theory and nursing practice', *Journal of Advanced Nursing*, 1: 414–24.

—— (1989), 'Theory to practice: implementation in the clinical setting', in Jolley, M. and Allen, P. (eds), *Current Issues in Nursing*, London: Chapman & Hall.

Minshull, J., Ross, K. and Turner, J. (1986), 'The human needs model of nursing', *Journal of Advanced Nursing*, 11: 643–9.

Mishel, M.H. (1990), 'Reconceptualisation of the uncertainty in illness theory', *Image: The Journal of Nurse Scholarship*, 22: 256–61.

Mitchell, R.G. (1986), *Essential Psychiatric Nursing*, Edinburgh: Churchill Livingstone.

Moody, L.E. (1990), *Advancing Nursing Science through Research* (Vol. 1). Newbury Park: Sage.

Moody, L.E., Wilson, M., Smyth, K., Schwartz, R., Tittle, M. and VanCott, M. (1988), 'Analysis of a decade of nursing practice research', *Nursing Research*, 37: 374–9.

Morse, J.M. (1995), 'Exploring the theoretical basis of nursing using advanced techniques of concept analysis', *Advance in Nursing Science*, 17(3): 31–46.

Moscow, D. (1986), 'Effective implementation of organisational development in the NHS', *Health Services Manpower Review*, 12(2): 3–7.

Neuman, B. (1982), *The Neuman Systems Model: Application to Nursing Education and Practice*, Norwalk, Conn.: Appleton–Century–Crofts.

—— (1995), *The Neuman Systems Model* (3rd edn), Norwalk, Conn.: Appleton & Lange.

Neuman, B. and Young, R.J. (1972), 'A model for teaching total person approach to patient problems', *Nursing Research*, 21(3): 264.

Newell, R. (1992), 'Anxiety, accuracy and reflection: the limits of professional development', *Journal of Advanced Nursing*, 17(11): 1326–33.

Newman, M.A. (1979), *Theory Development in Nursing* (2nd edn), Philadelphia: F.A. Davis.

—— (1994), *Theory Development in Nursing* (3rd edn), Philadelphia: F.A. Davis.

Nicholl, L.H. (1992), *Perspectives on Nursing Theory* (2nd edn), Boston: Little Brown & Co. (reprinted from *Image* 9(3): 59–63).

Nightingale, F. (1859), *Notes on Nursing: What It Is and What It Is Not* (reprinted 1980), Edinburgh: Churchill Livingstone.

Nolan, P.W. (1989), 'Psychiatric nursing past and present: the nurses' viewpoint', unpublished Ph.D. thesis, University of Bath.

Norris, C.M. (1970), *Proceedings from the Second Annual Nursing Theory Conference*, Kansas: University of Kansas.

—— (1982), *Concept Clarification in Nursing*, Rockville: Aspen Systems Corp.

Nursing Theories Conference Group (1975), *Nursing Theories: The Base for Professional Practice* (Chairman, Julia George), Englewood Cliffs: Prentice Hall.

Nursing Theories Think-tank (1979), *Advances in Nursing Science*, 1(3): 105.

Openshaw, S. (1984), 'Clinical judgement by nurses: decision strategies and nurses' appraisal of patient affect', unpublished Ph.D. thesis, University of London.

Orem, D.E. (1959), *Guides for Development of Curriculae for the Education of Practical Nurses*, Washington D.C.: US Department of Health, Education and Welfare.

Orem, D.E. (1980), *Nursing: Concepts of Practice* (3rd edn), New York: McGraw Hill.

—— (1985), *Nursing: Concepts of Practice* (4th edn), New York: McGraw Hill.

—— (1995), *Nursing: Concepts of Practice* (5th edn), New York: McGraw Hill.

Orlando, I. (1961), *The Dynamic Nurse–Patient Relationship: Function, Process, and Principles*, New York: G.P. Putnam & Sons.

Orr, J. (1992), 'The pathway to quality care', presentation at Northern Ireland National Board's Annual Conference, Belfast, NINB, October.

Parker, J. (1991), 'Being and nature: an interpretation of person and environment', in Gray, G. and Pratt, R. (eds), *Towards a Discipline of Nursing*, Edinburgh: Churchill Livingstone.

Parse, R.R. (1981), *Man–Living–Health: A Theory of Nursing*, New York: Wiley & Sons.

—— (1987), *Nursing Science: Major Paradigms, Theories and Critiques*, Philadelphia: W.B. Saunders.

—— (1993), 'Response to theory guides research and practice', *Nursing Science Quarterly*, 6(1): 12.

—— (1995), *Illuminations: The Human Becoming Theory in Practice and Research*, New York: NLN.

Parsons, T. (1952), *The Social System*, London: Tavistock.

Patterson, J.G. and Zderad, L.T. (1976), *Humanistic Nursing*, New York: John Wiley & Sons.

Pearson, A. (1985), 'The effects of introducing new norms in a nursing unit and an analysis of the process of change', unpublished Ph.D. thesis, University of London.

—— (1986), 'Nursing models and multidisciplinary teamwork', in Kershaw, B. and Salvage, J. (eds), *Models for Nursing*, Chichester: John Wiley & Sons.

Pearson, A. and Vaughan, B. (1986), *Nursing Models for Practice*, London: Heinemann.

Peplau, H.E. (1952), *Interpersonal Relations in Nursing*, New York: G.P. Putnam & Sons.

—— (1987), 'Nursing science: a historical perspective', in Parse, R.R. (ed.), *Nursing Science: Major Paradigms, Theories and Critiques*, Philadelphia: W.B. Saunders.

Peplau, H.E. (1995), 'Schizophrenia', conference presentation, Annual Conference of Nursing, University of Ulster, Northern Ireland.

Perkins, J. (1965), cited in Hoon, E. (1986), 'Game playing: a new way to look at models', *Journal of Advanced Nursing*, 11: 421–7.

Pierce, C.S. (1957), *Essays in the Philosophy of Science*, Indianapolis: Bobbs-Merrill.

Polanyi, M. (1958), *Personal Knowledge*, Chicago: University of Chicago Press.

Polit, D. and Hungler, B. (1983), *Nursing Research: Principles and Methods* (2nd edn), Philadelphia: Lippincott.

Popper, K. (1965), *Conjectures and Refutations: The Growth of Scientific Knowledge*, New York: Harper & Row.

Powers, B.A. and Knapp, T.R. (1995), *A Dictionary of Nursing Theory and Research* (2nd edn), Newbury Park: Sage.

Rafferty, A.M., Allcock, N. and Lathlean, J. (1996), 'The theory–practice gap: taking issue with the issue', *Journal of Advanced Nursing*, 23(4): 685–91.

Rambo, B.J. (1984), *Adaptation Nursing: Assessment and Intervention*, Philadelphia: W.B. Saunders.

Reed, P.G. (1987), 'Constructing a conceptual framework for psychosocial nursing', *Journal of Psychosocial Nursing*, 25(2): 24–8.

—— (1989), 'Nursing theorizing as an ethical endeavour', *Advances in Nursing Science*, 11(3): 1–9.

Reynolds, P.D. (1971), *A Primer for Theory Construction*, Indianapolis: Bobbs-Merrill.

Rhyl, G. (1963), *The Concept of the Mind*, London: Penguin.

Riehl, J.P. (1974), 'The Riehl interactional model', in Riehl, J.P. and Roy, C. (eds), *Conceptual Models for Nursing Practice*, New York: Appleton–Century–Crofts.

Riehl, J.P. and Roy, C. (1980), *Conceptual Models for Nursing Practice* (2nd edn; 1st edn 1974), New York: Appleton–Century–Crofts.

Roach, M.S. (1984), *Caring: The Human Mode of Being: Implications for Nursing*, Toronto: University of Toronto, Faculty of Nursing.

—— (1992), 'The aim of philosophical inquiry in nursing: unity or diversity of thought?', in Kikuchi, J.F. and Simmons, H. (eds), *Philosophic Inquiry in Nursing*, Newbury Park: Sage.

Robinson, J.A. (1992), 'Problems with paradigms in a caring profession', *Journal of Advanced Nursing*, 17: 632–8.

—— (1994), 'Problems with paradigms in a caring profession', in Smith, J.P. (ed.), *Models, Theories and Concepts*, Oxford: Blackwell Scientific Press.

Robinson, K. (1990), 'Nursing models: the hidden costs', *Surgical Nurse*, 3(7): 11–14.

Rodgers, B.L. (1994), 'Concepts, analysis and the development of nursing knowledge: the evolutionary cycle', in Smith, J.P. (ed.), *Models, Theories and Concepts*, Oxford: Blackwell Scientific Press.

Rogers, E. (1983), *Diffusion of Innovations*, New York: Free Press.

Rogers, J.A. (1974), 'Theoretical considerations involved in the process of change', in Backer, B.A., Dubbert, P.M. and Eisenman, E.J.P. (eds), *Psychiatric/Mental Health Nursing: Contemporary Readings*, New York: Van Nostrand.

Rogers, M.E. (1961), *Educational Revolution in Nursing*, New York: Macmillan.

—— (1970), *An Introduction to a Theoretical Basis of Nursing*, Philadelphia: F.A. Davis & Co.

—— (1980), *An Introduction to a Theoretical Basis of Nursing* (2nd edn), Philadelphia: F.A. Davis & Co.

—— (1990), *An Introduction to a Theoretical Basis of Nursing* (3rd edn), Philadelphia: F.A. Davis & Co.

Rogers, R. (1986), 'Choosing is taking a political stance', *Senior Nurse*, 5(4): 4.

Roper, N., Logan, N. and Tierney, A. (1983), *Using a Model for Nursing*, Edinburgh: Churchill Livingstone.

Roper, N., Logan, N. and Tierney, A. (1990), *Elements of Nursing*, (3rd edn; 1st edn 1980; 2nd edn 1985), Edinburgh: Churchill Livingstone.

Rosenbaum, J.N. (1986), 'Comparison of two theorists on care: Orem and Leininger', *Journal of Advanced Nursing*, 11: 409–19.

Rotter, J.B. (1966), 'Generalised expectancies for internal versus external control of reinforcement', *Psychological Monographs*, 80(1): 19–24.

Roy, C. (1970), 'Adaptation – a conceptual framework for nursing', *Nursing Outlook*, 18(3): 42–5.

Roy, C. (1971), 'Adaptation: a basis for nursing practice', *Nursing Outlook*, 19(4): 254–7.

—— (1980), 'The Roy adaptation model', in Riehl, J.P. and Roy, C. (eds), *Conceptual Models for Nursing Practice* (2nd edn), New York: Appleton–Century–Crofts.

—— (1989), 'Nursing care in theory and practice: early interventions in brain injury', in Harris, R., Burns, R. and Rees, R. (eds), *Recovery from Brain Injury*, Adelaide: Institute for the Study of Learning Difficulties.

—— (1996), *The Roy Adaptation Model: The Definitive Statement*, Norwalk, Conn.: Appleton & Lange.

Salanders, L. and Dietz-Omar, M. (1991), 'Making nursing models relevant for the practising nurse', *Nursing Practice*, 4(2): 23–5.

Salsberry, P.J. (1994), 'A philosophy of nursing: what it is and what it is not', in Kikuchi, J.F. and Simmons, H. (eds), *Developing a Philosophy of Nursing*, Newbury Park: Sage.

Salvage, J. (1990), 'Introduction', in Salvage, J. and Kershaw, B. (eds), *Models of Nursing 2*, London: Scutari Press.

Sampson, E. (1971), *Social Psychology and Contemporary Science*, New York: John Wiley & Sons.

Sandelowski, M. (1993), 'Theory unmasked: the uses and guises of theory in qualitative research', *Research in Nursing and Health*, 16: 213–18.

Sarter, B. (1988), 'Philosophical sources of nursing theory', *Nursing Science Quarterly*, 1(2): 52–9.

—— (1991), 'Philosophical foundations of nursing theory', in Chaska, N. (ed.), *The Nursing Profession: Turning Points*, St Louis: C.V. Mosby.

Schein, E.H. (1969), *Organisational Psychology*, New Jersey: Prentice Hall.

Schlotfeldt, R.M. (1992), 'Answering nursing's philosophical questions: whose responsibility is it?', in Kikuchi, J.F. and Simmons, H. (eds), *Philosophic Inquiry in Nursing*, Newbury Park: Sage.

Schmieding, N. (1990), 'An integrative nursing theoretical framework', *Journal of Advanced Nursing*, 15: 463–7.

Schon, D. (1987), *Educating the Reflective Practitioner*, San Francisco: Jossey Bass.

Seligman, M. (1971), 'Fall into helplessness', *Psychology Today*, 7: 43–8.

Sharp, T. (1991), 'Whose problem?', *Nursing Times*, 87(3): 36–8.

Silva, M.C. (1977), 'Philosophy, science, theory: interrelationships and implications for nursing research', *Image: The Journal of Nurse Scholarship*, 9(3): 59–63.

—— (1986a), 'Philosophy, science, theory: interrelationships and implications for nursing research', in Nicholl, L.H. (1992) (ed.), *Perspectives on Nursing Theory* (2nd edn), Boston: Little, Brown & Co. (reprinted from *Image* 9(3): 59–63).

—— (1986b), 'Research testing nursing theory: the state of the art', *Advances in Nursing Science*, 9(1): 1–11.

Slevin, O. (1995), 'Theories and models', in Bashford, P. and Slevin, O. (eds), *Theory and Practice in Nursing*, Edinburgh: Campion Press.

—— (1996), 'Theory, research and practice: towards a new praxis in nursing', unpublished manuscript, National Board for Nursing, Midwifery and Health Visiting, Belfast.

Smith, E.E. and Medin, D.L. (1981), *Categories and Concepts*, Cambridge, Mass.: Harvard University Press.

Smith, L. (1982), 'Models of nursing as the basis for curriculum development: some rationales and implications', *Journal of Advanced Nursing*, 7: 117–27.

—— (1986), 'Issues raised by the use of nursing models in psychiatry', *Nurse Education Today*, 6: 69–75.

—— (1987), 'Applications of a nursing model to a curriculum: some considerations', *Nurse Education Today*, 7: 109–15.

Smith, M.C. (1990), 'Knowledge development: pushing from within or pulling from without?', *Nursing Science Quarterly*. 2(4): 156.

—— (1994), 'Arriving at a philosophy of nursing: discovering? constructing? evolving?', in Kikuchi, J.F. and Simmons, H. (eds), *Developing a Philosophy of Nursing*, Newbury Park: Sage.

Smoyak, S. (1988), 'Knowledge is knowledge', paper presented at the Fifth Nursing Science Colloquium, Boston, Mass., Boston University School of Nursing.

Sorrentino, E. (1991), 'Making theories work for you', *Nursing Administration Quarterly*, 15: 54–9.

Speedy, S. (1989), 'Theory–practice debate: setting the scene', *Australian Journal of Advanced Nursing Practice*, 6(3): 12–20.

Sternberg, P. (1986), 'Models and theories have not changed practice', (letter), *Nursing Times*, 83(46): 12.

Stevens, B.J. (1979), *Nursing Theory: Analysis, Application, Evaluation* (1st edn), Boston: Little, Brown & Co.

Stevens-Barnum, B.J. (1994), *Nursing Theory: Analysis, Application, Evaluation* (4th edn), Philadelphia: Lippincott.

Stevenson, J. and Woods, N. (1985), cited in Sorenson, G. (ed.), *Setting the Agenda for the Year 2000: Knowledge Development in Nursing*, Kansas City, Mo.: ANA.

Stockwell, F. (1985), *The Nursing Process in Psychiatric Nursing*, London: Croom Helm.

Storch, J.L. (1986), 'In defence of nursing theory', *The Canadian Nurse*, 82(16): 16–20.

Suchman, E.A. (1967), *Evaluative Research*, New York: Russell Sage Foundation.

Sullivan, H.S. (1953), 'The interpersonal theory of psychiatry', in Perry, H.S. and Gawel, M.L. (eds), *Conceptions of Modern Psychiatry*, New York: W. W. Norton & Co.

Suppe, F. (1977), *The Structure of Scientific Theories* (2nd edn), Urbana: University of Illinois Press.

Suppe, F. and Jacox, A. (1985), 'Philosophy of science and the development of nursing theory', in Werley, H. and Fitzpatrick, J.J. (eds), *Annual Review of Nursing Research*, 3: 241–67.

Swanson, K.M. (1991), 'Empirical development of a mid-range theory of caring', *Nursing Research*, 40: 241–67.

Tierney, A. (1973), 'Toilet training', *Nursing Times*, 69: 1740–5.

Toffler, A. (1970), *Future Shock*, New York: Random House.

Toulmin, S. (1972), *Human Understanding*, Princeton: Princeton University Press.

Travelbee, J. (1966), *Interpersonal Aspects of Nursing*, Philadelphia: F.A. Davis.

Tversky, A. and Kahneman, D. (1981), 'The framing of decisions and the psychology of choice', *Science*, 211: 453–8.

Uys, L. (1987), 'Foundational studies in nursing', *Journal of Advanced Nursing*, 12: 275–80.

Vaughan, B. (1990), 'Knowing that and knowing how: the role of the lecturer-practitioner', in Salvage, J. and Kershaw, B. (eds), *Models for Nursing 2*, London: Scutari Press.

Vinokuv, A. (1971), 'Review and theoretical analysis of the effects of group processes upon individual and group decisions involving risk', *Psychological Bulletin*, 76: 231–50.

Von Bertalanffy, L. (1951), 'General systems theory: a new approach to unity of science', *Human Biology*, 121: 303–61.

Wald, F.S. and Leonard, R.C. (1964), 'Towards the development of nursing practice theory', *Nursing Research*, 13(4): 309–13.

Walker, L.O. (1971), 'Towards a clearer understanding of the concept of nursing theory', *Nursing Research*, 20(5): 428–35.

—— (1973), 'Theory, practice and research in perspective', in Nicholl, L. (1991) (ed.), *Perspectives on Nursing Theory* (2nd edn), New York: J.P. Lippincott.

Walker L.O. and Avant, K.C. (1983), *Strategies for Theory Construction in Nursing*, Norwalk, Conn.: Appleton & Lange.

Walker L.O. and Avant, K.C. (1995), *Strategies for Theory Construction in Nursing* (3rd edn), Norwalk, Conn.: Appleton & Lange.

Walsh, M. (1989), 'Model example', *Nursing Standard*, 22(3): 22–4.

—— (1990), 'From model to care plan', in Salvage, J. and Kershaw, B. (eds), *Models for Nursing 2*, London: Scutari Press.

—— (1991), *Models in Clinical Nursing: The Way Forward*, London: Baillière Tindall.

Watson, J. (1973), *A Model of Caring: An Alternative Health Care Model for Nursing Practice and Research* (1st edn), New York: American Nurses Association (Pub. no. NP-59 3M 8179190).

—— (1979), *A Model of Caring: An Alternative Health Care Model for Nursing Practice and Research* (2nd edn), New York: American Nurses Association (Pub. no. NP-59 3M 8179190).

—— (1985), *Nursing: Human Science and Care*, New York: Appleton–Century–Crofts.

Webb, C. (1984), 'On the eighth day God created the nursing process and nobody rested!' *Senior Nurse*, 1(33): 22–5.

—— (1986a), 'Organising care, nursing models: a personal view', *Nursing Practice*, 1: 208–12.

—— (ed.) (1986b), *Using Nursing Models Series: Women's Health, Midwifery and Gynaecological Nursing*, London: Hodder & Stoughton.

Wewers, M.A. and Lenz, E.R. (1987), 'Relapse among ex-smokers:

an example of theory derivation', *Advances in Nursing Science*, 9(2): 44–53.

Whall, A. (1989), 'The influence of logical positivism on nursing practice', *Image: The Journal of Nurse Scholarship*, 21: 243–5.

Whitehead, A.N. (1933), *The Aims of Education*, London: Benn.

Wiedenbach, E. (1964), *Clinical Nursing: A Helping Art*, New York: Springer.

Williams, C.A. (1979), 'The nature and development of conceptual frameworks', in Downs, F.S. and Fleming, J.W. (eds), *Issues in Nursing Research*, New York: Appleton–Century–Crofts.

Wilson, J. (1969), *Thinking with Concepts*, London: Cambridge University Press.

Wood, C. (1880), *A Handbook of Nursing for the Home and the Hospital*, London: Cassell.

Woodham-Smith, C.B. (1977), *Florence Nightingale 1820–1910*, London: Collins.

Wooldridge, P.J. (1992), 'The author comments', in Nicholl, L.H. (ed.), *Perspectives on Nursing Theory* (2nd edn), Philadelphia: J.B. Lippincott.

Wright, S.G. (1985), 'It's all right in theory', *Nursing Times*, 81(34): 19–20.

—— (1986), *Building and Using a Model of Nursing*, London: Edward Arnold.

—— (1988), 'Debate 1: this house believes that nursing models provide a useful tool in the management of patient care', in Pritchard, A.P. (ed.), *Proceedings of the Fifth International Conference on Cancer Nursing*, London: Macmillan Press.

Yoo, K.H. (1991), 'Expectation and evaluation of occupational health nursing services, as perceived by occupational health nurses, employees and employers in the United Kingdom', unpublished Ph.D. thesis, University of Ulster.

Yura, H. and Torres, G. (1975), 'Today's conceptual frameworks within baccalaureate nursing programs', in *Faculty-Curriculum Development. Part III: Conceptual Framework, its Meaning and Function*, New York: National League of Nursing (Pub. no. 15–1558.

Zaltman, G. and Duncan, R. (1977), *Strategies for Planned Change*, New York: John Wiley & Sons.

Index